Breastfeeding
Twins and Triplets

of related interest

Supporting Breastfeeding Past the First Six Months and Beyond
A Guide for Professionals and Parents
Emma Pickett
ISBN 978 1 78775 989 3
eISBN 978 1 78775 990 9

Supporting Queer Birth
A Book for Birth Professionals and Parents
AJ Silver
ISBN 978 1 83997 045 0
eISBN 978 1 83997 046 7

Supporting Autistic Women through Pregnancy and Childbirth
Hayley Morgan, Emma Durman and Dr Alys Einion-Waller
ISBN 978 1 83997 105 1
eISBN 978 1 83997 106 8

Weaving the Cradle
Facilitating Groups to Promote Attunement and Bonding
between Parents, Their Babies and Toddlers
Edited by Monika Celebi
Foreword by Jane Barlow
ISBN 978 1 84819 311 6
eISBN 978 0 85701 264 7

Breastfeeding Twins and Triplets

A Guide for Professionals and Parents

Kathryn Stagg

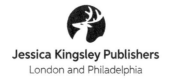

Jessica Kingsley Publishers
London and Philadelphia

First published in Great Britain in 2023 by Jessica Kingsley Publishers
An imprint of Hodder & Stoughton Ltd
An Hachette Company

1

The information contained in this book is not intended to replace the services of trained
medical professionals or to be a substitute for medical advice. You are advised to consult a
doctor on any matters relating to your health, and in particular on any matters that may
require diagnosis or medical attention.

A CIP catalogue record for this title is available from the British Library and the Library
of Congress

ISBN 978 1 83997 049 8
eISBN 978 1 83997 050 4

Printed and bound by CPI Group (UK) Ltd, Croydon, CR0 4YY

Jessica Kingsley Publishers' policy is to use papers that are natural, renewable, and
recyclable products and made from wood grown in sustainable forests. The logging and
manufacturing processes are expected to conform to the environmental regulations of
the country of origin.

Jessica Kingsley Publishers
Carmelite House
50 Victoria Embankment
London EC4Y 0DZ

www.jkp.com

Contents

Acknowledgements

I do not actually know where to start with thanking people, so I am going to start at the very beginning with my mum! I was always brought up knowing I could do anything and that she would support me. She was also a huge support for me in the early days of my own breastfeeding and parenting journey. She also knew it was my journey and that I needed to find my own way. And my partner Darren for supporting me to breastfeed and for understanding that it was important to me. And to my own journey, this book would not have happened if I had not been supported to breastfeed my own twins.

From the bank midwife on day 2 that showed me how to tandem feed (I wish I knew her name), to my community midwife Penny Estall, to Tracy Whaley who ran Harrow Twins Club Baby Group, and had also breastfed her twins, to Alison Spiro who ran our local breastfeeding group and later gave me the opportunity to train as a peer supporter – I volunteered beside her for 11 years, a true mentor. Catriona Hart for being that friend breastfeeding triplets so how could I give up just having two babies? Anne Murphy for being that friend round the corner I could have a moan and a cuppa with and we still do 17 years on. And Helen Wall, who kept telling me I should write a book! I set up the Breastfeeding Twins and Triplets UK Facebook group in 2015, so I want to send a big shout out to all the admins past and present who have helped make this such a wonderful corner of the internet: Tamsin, Jennie, Debra J, Debra R, Sarah H-J, Sarah M, Anna, Livvy, Nicki, Kim, Jennifer, Katie, Annie, Lucy and Cate, and the biggest shout out to Catherine Wakely who has been my right-hand woman throughout and also is a trained proofreader so made sure that the book made sense!

Also, a big shout out to our charity trustees, Ruth, Catherine, Ffion, Nicola, Katie, Kirsty our admin, and Jan Bonar who single-handedly (almost) made us think it was possible. And from the lactation world, Emma Pickett for suggesting I should write this and putting my name forward. Karen Kerkhoff Gromada for being my inspiration, her book *Mothering Multiples* was my bible. Tez Clark, Sophie Burrows, and Lucy Ruddle for listening to my worries. Miriam Feen for being my work other half and person I turn to for support. Thanks to Jessica Kingsley Publishers for giving me the opportunity and especially Maddy Budd. And thank you to all the parents I have supported over the years. You have taught me so much.

Notes on the text

This book is written from the perspective of breastfeeding multiples in the UK. All quotes given by parents were shared with the author in written form in 2020/2021 and consent was given for publication.

I support all families to meet their feeding goals, no matter how they look. Not all multiple birth families use the terms 'mother' and 'breastfeeding'. I have chosen to use the word 'breastfeeding' in this text but acknowledge some may prefer the term 'nursing' or 'chest-feeding'. I have also chosen to use the term 'breastfeeding parent' but acknowledge some would prefer to use 'mother'. All members of the babies' family are part of this journey. Families do indeed breastfeed.

This book is for information and is not intended to replace a breastfeeding consultation, diagnosis, or medical treatment from a qualified breastfeeding supporter, physician, or health care provider.

Chapter 1

Pregnancy – Discovering There Is More Than One

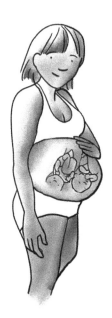

How do multiple births happen?

Twin pregnancies come in various forms. They can start from two eggs and two sperm fertilised separately – these babies will be as genetically alike as two standard siblings, and are known as fraternal twins. They just happen to be born on the same day. Each embryo will have their own separate placenta and amniotic sac, so this type of pregnancy is often referred to as DCDA (di-chorionic, di-amniotic).

Twins can also start from one egg fertilised by one sperm which, for reasons we do not understand, then splits into two separate, genetically identical, embryos. The time from fertilisation to division controls how separated the two embryos are. If a split occurs one to three days after fertilisation each baby will have their own sac and own placenta. This pregnancy will also be referred to as DCDA, so if parents have a DCDA pregnancy their babies could be fraternal or identical. If the split happens four to eight days after fertilisation the resulting embryos will be sharing a placenta but still have separate sacs. This is known as MCDA (mono-chorionic, di-amniotic). If the split happens 8 to 13 days after fertilisation, this results in the embryos sharing a placenta and also sharing a sac, known as MCMA (mono-chorionic, mono-amniotic).

If the split happens after 13 days this can result in conjoined twins (Jha, Morgan & Kennedy 2019). Conjoined twins do not separate completely and can still share some body parts and organs – though thankfully this is very rare.

Triplet pregnancies can start from three eggs and three sperm, resulting in three fraternal babies with separate sacs and placentas. They can be from two eggs and two sperm where one of the embryos splits, resulting in an identical pair and one fraternal baby. The identical pair can be DCDA, MCDA, or MCMA. Or, rarely, all three babies can be identical, the original embryo splitting twice into three babies.

DCDA pregnancies are the least risky of any multiple birth pregnancy. Normally parents are offered monthly scans and are generally more likely to be able to go into spontaneous labour and birth vaginally without complications. MCDA and MCMA pregnancies are higher risk so parents are often offered fortnightly scans, and babies tend to be delivered a little earlier and in a more medicalised way due to the risks of Twin to Twin Transfusion Syndrome (TTTS). MCMA babies are generally born by caesarean section due to the risk of their cords being entangled.

Discovering the news

Most families nowadays find out they are expecting a multiple birth at their first scan. This is generally around the 12 week point of pregnancy, although those going through fertility treatment often have an early scan to check all is ok. Before sonography, families often had no warning that there might be more than one baby until the actual birth. The first baby was born, and contractions started up again and another popped out – and sometimes even a third! Sometimes they had an inkling because their size did not match their dates, or their midwife could feel too many body parts.

However, multiple birth pregnancies are higher risk. The *MBRRACE-UK 2021 Perinatal Confidential Enquiry: Stillbirths and Neonatal Deaths in Twin Pregnancies* found that for twin pregnancies there is almost double the risk of stillbirth and over three times the risk of neonatal death compared to singleton pregnancies. In order to prevent this they suggest parents should be cared for by a specialist twin clinic, given a schedule of appointments and scans, and be educated in what to look out for if they go into early labour. However, the BeCOME research from Twins Trust found that 61% of the parents surveyed had no complications in pregnancy and 31% had one complication, with the most common issues being pre-eclampsia, Twin to Twin Transfusion Syndrome (MC pregnancies only), selective fetal growth restriction, threatened preterm birth before 28 weeks, and pregnancy induced diabetes (Twins Trust 2020).

Finding out in early pregnancy also gives parents some time to get used to the idea before the babies actually arrive. Expecting more than one baby is often a massive shock, and the news can trigger a huge range of emotions, some of which can be quite unexpected. Feelings can range from happiness, ecstasy, and relief, through to worry, grief, and devastation. If there have been fertility issues there can be a massive sense of relief, not only that the pregnancy is developing, but also that this one pregnancy will provide an 'instant family' and they may not need to go through the fertility process again to 'complete their family'. For others, having two babies at once can seem a total disaster. Many parents have planned their families. They may have wanted two children and their second pregnancy is twins. They may have had an unplanned pregnancy and now there are two babies. They may already have children from other relationships and now find themselves expecting triplets! All sorts of scenarios. There can be grief for the pregnancy they had planned, grief for the home birth they had envisaged, grief for the breastfeeding journey they wanted. The financial implications of expecting multiples are a common worry: maybe their house or car is too small, and of course there will be double the childcare costs.

And then there are the comments expectant parents often get from friends and family, and from health care professionals!

'How will you cope?'
'Rather you than me!'
'Twins would be my worst nightmare!'
'Double Trouble!'
'I always wanted twins...until I had one baby!'
'My sister/aunt/cousin/hairdresser had twins and it was so hard.'
'Of course, you will have to have a caesarean.'
'Of course, they will come early.'
'You won't make enough milk for more than one baby.'
'Of course, you won't be able to breastfeed...'

Expectant parents are already having to deal with their own worries about this multiple birth situation, but also have to deal with other people's reactions, which are not always encouraging!

Antenatal care

Positive antenatal conversations can help parents understand and feel more confident to take control of their pregnancy and birth and establish breastfeeding. It is very easy to feel that there is no choice around birth, and it is often suggested that families opt for a medicalised, controlled birth at a certain gestation. While there is a lot of evidence that there are optimal times to birth a multiple pregnancy, it is important that families do their research, ask for the reasons why these suggestions are being given and agree to a plan where everybody is happy. Parents should be encouraged to explore the research, the National Institute for Health and Care Excellence (NICE) guidelines and make an informed decision based on their own situation.

Multiple birth families are offered more antenatal appointments and scanned more frequently to check the growth and health of the babies, and to pick up any complications that may occur. DCDA parents should be offered eight appointments during pregnancy; MCDA and higher order multiples are offered more, as risks are higher.

Around 60% of twin pregnancies result in spontaneous labour before 37 weeks, and 75% of triplet pregnancies result in spontaneous labour before 35 weeks. In the UK parents with uncomplicated DCDA pregnancies will be offered a planned birth from 37 weeks, and uncomplicated MCDA pregnancies offered a planned birth from 36 weeks, as this does not appear to increase the risk of serious neonatal outcomes. However, there are implications to breastfeeding outcomes with births at this gestation, as we will discuss later. This birth plan can be declined, and in this scenario parents should be offered weekly appointments and scans (NICE 2019). The risks and benefits of antenatal corticosteroids and timings should be discussed in relation to lung development for preterm babies and delayed lactogenesis II (a delay in the mature milk 'coming in') (Henderson *et al.* 2008).

The implications to milk production and establishing breastfeeding should always be considered alongside other risks to morbidity and mortality when discussing birth interventions, timing and medication. Breastfeeding factors are too often not mentioned, leaving parents unaware that these decisions can affect feeding outcomes.

Helping the parents to focus on what they can control by making a birth plan for different situations can help them to feel like they have more choices. Likewise, making a feeding plan for what they would wish to happen depending on the different birthing situations can help focus the parent on what happens after birth. It is a great time to prepare.

If there is a known risk of premature delivery, parents should be encouraged to visit the neonatal unit if possible. It can be quite a daunting place – all the wires, machines, noises, busy staff. Knowing what to expect and what everything means will help the parents to cope if they find themselves in this stressful situation.

PERSONAL STORIES
Matilde with Filippo and Tommaso

I did a pregnancy test at home as my period was late. The positive line appeared instantly, even before the control one. Yay I was pregnant! We were obviously really happy and started to plan the following steps.

We decided to book a private scan as we couldn't wait. For the two weeks leading up to the appointment my husband would constantly joke about having twins, saying, 'Hi babies' to my belly etc. We have twins in both our families but I always said, 'No please, one kid is enough to start with! We are alone here (our families are in Italy), let's just start with one!'

On the morning of the scan he said, 'Let's go and meet our babies.' The technician immediately found one baby, strong heartbeat, good position etc. We were so excited, emotional, almost crying with happiness. Then she stopped and said she might have to do an internal scan – I panicked. I knew these were done if there are problems with the pregnancy. She continued with the external scan and said, 'I thought it was my eyes playing a trick on me being early morning, but no, here you go, two babies!' And she managed to capture both in the same frame!

Our reaction? We burst out laughing! She definitely didn't expect that, she actually looked a bit shocked! We couldn't stop laughing, but I managed to explain about my husband's prediction and she laughed with us. We calmed down so she could check the second baby, again strong heartbeat etc.

We were obviously over the moon!

Caroline with Alexander and William

I found out I was pregnant quite early on. My partner and I had been trying to conceive for six months, so I was paying more attention to my body than usual. I ended up testing the day my period was due. The test was positive, so I booked in a doctor's appointment. We were sent for a scan. I remember the sonographer just going quiet and looking at me. Panicked, I looked at the screen. I work as a veterinarian and so have some experience reading ultrasounds, and straight away I suspected what was going on.

'Oh my god is there two?! There's two, isn't there?' I said. When she nodded, I swore and burst into tears. Although my partner was very keen for a family, I wasn't even sure I liked children, and had barely come around to the idea of having one, let alone two! I was in shock, and very, very anxious about the prospect.

Jana with Isla and Anya (first set) and River and Raine (second set)

Wow, a second set of twins, what a blessing, we would hear. So why did I feel such an overwhelming amount of fear and a slight twang of regret. I remember being stuck between the highest of emotions and the worrying reality of what was to come. I think it's easier when you know nothing other than more than one baby, like when my first set of twins were born in 2009. Here I was, 12 years later, having had a singleton in 2016, knowing exactly what was to come. This in itself came with a range of emotions including guilt for even feeling this way. Who am I to complain when many women struggle to even have just one child? As time went on I truly did accept our double, double blessing, but it absolutely was ok to explore those initial feelings of doubt and anxieties. Allowing myself to speak to my partner openly about my feelings meant we could work through the doubts and have ended up excited and prepared, physically and mentally. There will be worries, along with pure happiness and excitement and it's all absolutely normal and ok.

Keri with Billie-Ray, Herbie, and Stanley

On the day of my scan I had to go alone, due to the infection control rules at that time, but I was excited. We'd decided to have a third baby, to finish off our family nicely, and this was the first time I had a nice baby bump. With my first two I just looked a bit fat until I was seven or eight months. So I happily went along feeling nice and pregnant!

During my scan I looked at the screen and thought I could see two babies, but what do I know! After a few minutes my sonographer said 'well...' and I interrupted with 'Oh god! It's not twins is it!?' and she said, 'No, it's not twins but I do see triplets!' she then showed me three heartbeats and left me, to go and get another sonographer. After that I had the rest of my scan which took around 45 minutes and I literally switched between crying and laughing hysterically. I couldn't believe it! As soon as I left the room and I was waiting for my partner to come and get me I just started to panic. Like how was I going to have three babies, at the same time!? What about the car, we live in a two-bed terrace, and then feeding! It just felt like the most impossible thing.

As my partner pulled up this weird fear of telling him covered me. I was worried about his reaction and what if he panicked. I felt like we couldn't both panic! He commented on how it was nice to be given so many pictures. That's when I just said 'There's three babies' and he looked at me like I was speaking a foreign language. I pointed at one picture and explained that was two babies in the same sac and I'd been told they'd be identical. Then I pointed to the other baby and explained they had their own sac and that made three. He took the news really well, feeling that it was crazy but exciting. I, meanwhile, not so much! Not only did I not want triplets, I didn't want five kids in total. Honestly, I took pretty much my entire pregnancy to get happy about this, and even then I don't think I was happy – I think I'd just come to terms with it. But eventually, probably mainly once they'd actually been born, I realised this wasn't their fault or in their control any more than it was in ours. I felt guilty for being so unhappy about this pregnancy, especially as we'd planned it. But at the same time this wasn't what I'd planned... Now, though, I just couldn't imagine our family any other way. It's been crazy and hard and plain daft at times, but I'm glad I'm in the club!

Parents that are already breastfeeding

Some parents fall pregnant while they are still breastfeeding their previous child. One study shows that you are nine times more likely to fall pregnant with twins if you are breastfeeding (Steinman 2001). Although a multiple pregnancy is higher risk than a singleton pregnancy, there is a need for more research. Data suggest that breastfeeding during singleton pregnancy does not affect the way pregnancies end, or even birth weights (López-Fernández *et al.* 2017).

Hilary Flower states in her book *Adventures in Tandem Nursing*:

> If there is indeed added risk for twin pregnancies overlapping with breastfeeding, only direct study will be able to say for sure. The answer may vary greatly depending on the individual situations. We do know that some mothers do continue nursing and have healthy babies at term, based on mothers contributing to this book and one case study. (Flower 2019, p.49)

When pregnant and breastfeeding, some parents find they experience unmanageable levels of pain and aversion, while others are not affected by these symptoms at all. Milk production tends to reduce around the beginning of the second trimester. Some toddlers will wean when this happens, others do not seem to mind and continue to nurse anyway. If the older sibling is still of an age where milk is the majority of their diet, alternative milk may be necessary. In the latter part of the second trimester colostrum production begins, and if toddlers have dry-nursed through this period they are then able to have this colostrum.

Once the babies arrive it is possible to continue breastfeeding the older sibling as well. It is important to prioritise the needs of the new babies as they are solely dependent on the milk of their mother, but toddlers can be useful to help with clearing any engorgement or blocked ducts, and also to increase milk production. Some parents find that this is unsustainable or they can experience aversion to the older sibling feeding, but for others it works well and they can continue to breastfeed all with no issues.

There are no easy answers. Each parent must make their own evaluation of the benefits and risks of their own situation.

PERSONAL STORY
Lilli with Bowie and Camden

Not one to do things by half, I was very fortunate to conceive in February 2017. With an already 18-month-old and just turned three-year-old nurslings, I was very aware of the forthcoming task ahead. I realised that this pregnancy and the changes in milk taste could lead to my eldest and possibly my (now) middle child's end to their breastfeeding journey. Though, equally, I had already fed throughout one pregnancy and managed (purely by the grace of hormones) to maintain supply. I could do it again couldn't I? I have no idea how to parent without breasts. I nursed them both to sleep and transferred them to their beds. Tantrums, toothache, bumps and falls, were all solved with boob. Yup, I now thought of how I was going to do all that with number three in my arms too!

Time came around to the 12 week scan. The sonographer flits the camera over my belly back and forth, my husband and I staring up and the screen holding our breath. He turns to me, his eyes sparkled and he said, 'Which one do you want to see first?' And there you have it – the moment we realised we were now a family of six.

My supply dipped around 22–26 weeks, my eldest said the milk tasted like strawberries but that there wasn't much (handy when they can articulate to you exactly what is going on isn't it?). My younger one would latch and get bored from wasted effort at the measly offerings. But the three of us stuck with it, through dry nursing, hormonal nipple pain and taste changes.

The twins arrived after a speedy delivery and required some support in hospital. Here I was in hospital, with two babies who weren't able to nurse directly, pumping and hand expressing for them around the clock. I became engorged when my milk finally came in. Bless those toddlers! They swooped in to my rescue at visiting time. Although tender to touch, the relief from my older two drawing out the blocked milk from my inflamed ducts was awesome. For this reason alone, continuing to nurse them throughout pregnancy was well worth it.

While the twins were tiny, their little mouths and shallow latches meant their effectiveness at milk transfer was limited. Thankfully, I had a couple of useful toddlers to help establish my supply! In hospital I'd been advised to use the hospital grade double pump, and power pump as much as possible. With this in mind, by tandem feeding one of my older two with one of the twins, the let-down was brought on in both breasts, reducing the energy the breastfeeding twin required to use and increasing the milk they received. Every bit of stimulus my breasts received worked towards increasing the supply to service the twins. Some medical professionals were confused about the science of breastfeeding and felt my older two would be 'taking the milk from the babies' – but I knew and valued the importance of demand = supply = demand = supply. In the long run the twins' strength and latch would mature enough for them to manage and feed independently. For those initial weeks of learning, having this inclusive way of feeding I'm sure was fundamental to our overall success, as well as minimising any negative impact that can be experienced when introducing a newborn into the family, and transitioning siblings to their new 'big brother' or 'big sister' role.

Chapter 2

Preparing to Breastfeed

Learn about feeding

It is really important to learn about feeding before the babies arrive. You would not learn to drive just as you were heading down the slip road onto the motorway, and it's the same with breastfeeding. Its important parents do not leave it until the babies are actually born before learning how it works. Yes, breastfeeding is natural, but it is also a learned skill and it is important that parents have some knowledge of what is involved, and understand how to know whether the babies are feeding well and getting enough milk.

There may be an antenatal breastfeeding session at their local hospital or in the community. Or they may decide to do an online version so they can learn in the comfort of their own home. There are also multiple birth charities and social media groups that offer specialist 'breastfeeding multiples' webinars, live sessions, and the opportunity to witness others' experiences, as well as lots of great video tutorials online for singletons. After all, multiple birth babies are just babies, it's just that there are more of them! Second time parents who have already breastfed may need a refresher or may just want to learn about the specific barriers to breastfeeding of a multiple birth.

Milk production

Breasts begin making colostrum from sometime around half way through pregnancy, in a process called Lactogenesis I. Colostrum production is a bit like driving a car with the handbrake on. The breasts have all the power to make a full milk supply, but it is being restricted by the pregnancy hormone, progesterone, because there is no reason to make a full milk supply until there is a baby. Colostrum is the perfect food for babies in the first 48 hours or so, delivered in small quantities ideal for the babies' tiny tummies. It is rich in immunological components and prebiotics which may protect against bacteria and viruses and establish the early gut microbiome (Lawrence & Lawrence 2021).

Once the placenta is birthed, progesterone levels drop quite quickly and the handbrake comes off. The drop in progesterone allows levels of prolactin, the milk making hormone, to start to rise. This is called Lactogenesis ll. Generally milk increases in volume from around 30–40 hours after birth, but the parents often will not feel they are making more milk until two to three days after birth, or even later.

These first two stages of lactation are hormonally driven by the endocrine system. They occur whether or not the birthing parent is breastfeeding their baby.

Around nine to ten days after the birth of the placenta, milk production changes from being hormonally driven to being controlled by removal of the milk, using the autocrine system. This is known as Lactogenesis lll. Milk production is driven by baby feeding at the breast, or if baby cannot feed or is feeding inefficiently, a pump can be used to recreate this. It works on a supply and demand basis and frequency of breast stimulation is key – the more frequently the milk is removed, the more milk is made.

Returning to our driving analogy, at around six weeks postpartum, if all has been going well, milk production should be maintaining a nice motorway-style cruising speed, easily making what the babies require. This is when we say milk supply is 'established'.

There are sometimes difficulties in establishing a full milk supply, so parents have a bumpier road to navigate to reach full milk production. If they are not making a full milk supply by six weeks this does not mean it will not be possible to increase production. As the babies begin to feed more efficiently, or the parents begin to pump more frequently, there is often continuing potential to increase milk production. Six weeks is not a cut-off point in my experience.

Although we understand that stimulating the breasts frequently and efficiently in the early days is incredibly important to encourage full milk production by priming the prolactin receptor sites (De Carvalho *et al.* 1983), there seems to be little research as to whether there is a point when it can no longer be increased. After all, parents who have stopped breastfeeding completely (or even never started), can in fact, with support, re-lactate and make a full supply.

Breasts are a factory, not a warehouse. This is one of the common phrases in breastfeeding support. But what does it mean? Well, it means that every time milk is removed from the breast, production increases to replace it. Breasts are not a storage facility like a warehouse. They do not have a set amount of milk that they can provide. Breasts are a factory. Even during a feed, breasts are continually producing milk in the background. They are producing milk all the time, 24 hours a day. Prolactin is like the factory's workers, and is stimulated by a baby sucking at the breast. Prolactin levels rise in response to the suckling, and the more frequent the feeds the higher the levels of prolactin. These frequent feeds prevent a decline in of the concentration of prolactin before the next feed, and so production is maintained (Tay, Glasier & McNeilly 1996). Feeding two babies simultaneously has been shown to double the prolactin surge (Tyson *et al.* 1972).

There is another hormone active in breastfeeding which is very important: oxytocin. Oxytocin is stimulated by baby latching onto the breast, by skin to skin contact, by feeling safe and secure, and triggers a 'let-down' of milk, called the milk ejection reflex. The baby latching onto the breast triggers a surge of oxytocin, which squeezes the milk down into the breast by contracting the myoepithelial cells, forcing the milk into the ducts and making it available to the baby. This process delivers the milk which has been made by the prolactin fuelled milk making cells. The baby then draws out the milk by feeding efficiently at the breast. Oxytocin also causes the uterus to contract, helping to control post-partum bleeding. It encourages a feeling of calm in both parent and child, and plays an important role in the development of the attachment between infants and parents (Scatliffe *et al.* 2019).

If the babies need more milk they will feed more frequently. This causes more frequent surges in prolactin and oxytocin, and milk production will increase in response. If the babies take less milk then supply will reduce. If the babies are sleepy or not feeding very efficiently, or perhaps are fed on a strict schedule, or are given milk from another source like a bottle, then milk is left in the breast. In this situation, the mechanism called the feedback inhibitor of lactation tells the milk making cells they don't need to produce as much milk, and the body reduces production. Going back to our factory – if the babies feed less frequently, some of the workers are laid off and production falls. More research is needed on how this mechanism works.

So the key to milk production is frequent and efficient removal of the milk. If the babies are not breastfeeding well, pumping sessions may need to be added to establish a good milk supply. This is usually a temporary situation while the babies grow bigger and stronger and more able to fully breastfeed, or while breastfeeding support is found to work out how to help the babies breastfeed more efficiently.

Positioning baby at the breast

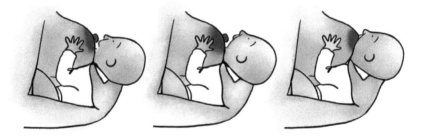

We often use the acronym CHINS to describe how to attach a baby to the breast.

C – CLOSE: Keep the baby close in to the adult's body, no matter which position they are feeding in. The baby's arms shouldn't be in the way, nor should there be any visible gap between baby's body and parent's body.

H – HEAD FREE: This means that nothing should prevent the baby being able to tip their head back in order to open their mouth wide. Sometimes the parent's arm, hand or a feeding cushion can get in the way of this – even a single finger on the back of the head can cause issues. Supporting the baby with a hand between the shoulder blades and fingers and thumb behind their ears supports baby's neck, but still allows them to put their head back to open wide.

I – IN LINE: The baby's body needs to be in a straight line to feed. So this means their ears, shoulders, and hips should all be lined up. If baby is having to turn sideways to feed then the whole baby should be turned to bring them into line.

N – NOSE TO NIPPLE: When preparing to feed, the baby should be lined up with the nipple just below their nose, and chin touching the breast. Tickling the baby's top lip with the nipple will stimulate their rooting reflex and baby should open their mouth wide. Baby can be brought onto the breast swiftly, leading with the chin.

S – SUSTAINABLE: The feeding position needs to be comfortable for the parent to sustain for a long period of time. Leaning back can help if the baby is feeding in an across the body position as this means gravity will help support the baby and keep them from slipping off the breast. For rugby hold (see Chapter 6) a good supportive cushion or cushions holding baby at the correct height to feed will make it sustainable.

It is important to take account of the parent's anatomy when positioning the baby. For example, if the parent has small, pert breasts with nipples pointing forward a baby feeding in cross cradle hold will need to be lying more on their side. Cross cradle hold is a popular position for single feeding, where the baby lies across the parent's body in a fairly horizontal position. If the parent has larger breasts with more downward pointing nipples, then baby will likely need to be lying more on their back to feed in cross cradle hold.

We need to make sure the nipple is pointing to the roof of baby's mouth. If you imagine an imaginary line coming out of the nipple it should point up to the roof of baby's mouth and out of the top of the back of baby's head. Baby's chin will be dug into the breast, and there will be a gap between nose and breast. Baby's body will be tucked close into the parent's body at the shoulders, with baby's arms around the breast.

It's also important to make sure baby is positioned so that both cheeks touch the breast equally at the sides. A baby who is offset is less likely to make a good seal, in which case the feed will be less efficient and they may take in more wind. So the breast should go into the mouth symmetrically, not pointing more towards the left or right of baby's head.

Larger breasts sound like they would be a good thing for breast-feeding twins or triplets, but actually they can make it quite difficult to achieve a deep latch. Large breasts tend to be very soft and malleable, and often the nipples point down, which can make it quite difficult for the parent to see what they are doing. Ideally, the parent will latch baby onto the breast where the breasts naturally fall – sometimes rugby hold works well for this as baby can lie on their back and be brought up to latch, and the breast tissue rests on baby's chest. A cradle hold with baby on their back can achieve a similar result.

However, sometimes the nipple is incredibly difficult for the parent to see, so there are a couple of tricks to try to make it easier. First rolling up a muslin, small towel, or blanket and placing it under the breast can raise it up and make the nipple more accessible. If this is not enough then taking a muslin square tied diagonally from corner to corner, or a scarf or other piece of fabric, and tying it around the parent's neck and under the breast can make a kind of breast sling. This lifts and supports the breast, making the nipple more accessible.

The pattern of a breastfeed

When the parent latches the baby onto the breast, the initial minute or so is taken up with fast, light sucks as the baby initiates the milk ejection reflex, or let-down. For some sleepy, early babies they will latch and then go quickly to sleep, as the milk flow is slow. Breast compressions can encourage these babies to suck and help stimulate the milk ejection reflex. Some babies can be quite fussy and come on and off the breast during this phase as they want a faster flow, and breast compressions can also help with this behaviour. After the milk ejection reflex, the milk is flowing and baby moves into a slower, deeper jaw motion, with long, rhythmic sucks and swallows with pauses every so often. We call this 'active feeding'. This is when baby is getting a good flow of milk and will take the majority of the feed. This active feeding can be of varying lengths depending on the efficiency of the baby, the flow of milk, the storage capacity of the parent, and the baby's size and stomach capacity. We cannot tell a parent that they must feed for a certain number of minutes as each dyad is completely unique. And, within a set of multiples, each baby can also be unique.

As the active feeding part comes to an end, baby moves into a lighter, more fluttery feeding pattern, with occasional swallows. The baby seems to be gently moving just their chin. They are still getting a little milk at this time and it is likely to be higher in fat. At the end of the feed the baby may wiggle and come off, or go to sleep and the nipple falls out of their mouth. But some babies can hang out all day comfort sucking, which is very inefficient! This can cause long feeds and make establishing breastfeeding, especially with more than one baby, tricky. Breast compressions can help them start the deeper sucking pattern again and sometimes they can trigger a second milk ejection, which causes baby to feed actively again. But if the breast compressions are not effective the parent can take the baby off. If baby stirs after a short time and wants to feed again, they can be put back onto the same breast. The baby will be awake and feeding more vigorously again, and so they will trigger another milk ejection reflex and will move back into the active feeding part of the feed again and take more milk. Human singleton babies are designed to feed on both breasts and are encouraged to do so in the early weeks. I suspect multiples also have this instinct. They often need more than one go on the breast to settle. I like to call it main course and pudding.

Normal newborn behaviour

It is incredibly important for all expectant parents to learn about normal newborn behaviour so they can prepare, and also understand when something is normal and when something needs to be investigated. For multiple birth families this is even more crucial. Just because their babies are twins or triplets does not mean they will behave differently from singletons. The challenge is how to deal with this as a parent when you have two or three of these newborns to deal with at once!

Babies like, and need, to feed frequently. One of the reasons for this is that the gastric half-emptying time for human milk is around 48 minutes (Cavkll 1981). Research into the stomach capacity of the newborn is not clear, but one study found that capacity is around 20mls, which translated as a feeding interval of around an hour for a term infant (Bergman 2013).

Some parents have larger or smaller milk storage capacity – although this has nothing to do with the size of the breasts. Some breasts contain more of the milk making tissue and so naturally store more milk. These differences do not make a difference to the parent's ability to breastfeed, except that those with a smaller storage capacity may find they need to offer a second go on the breast more frequently, or offer a feed a bit more often. A breast with a larger or smaller milk storage capacity will make enough milk for the babies as long as the parent follows their feeding cues. In an Australian study they found the average number of times a baby was fed to be 11 times in 24 hours, the range was 6 to 18 feeds, and the mother's milk storage capacity ranged from 74 to 382g per breast (Kent *et al.* 2006).

Another reason for a baby to feed frequently is that a baby's sleep cycle is around 50 minutes. They go from light sleep into deeper sleep, back into light sleep again, and then rouse. Sometimes parents may be able to encourage them to join two sleep cycles together with movement (buggy, car, sling, rocking etc.) or contact napping, but often it will take a feed to send them back to sleep. This frequent rousing is believed to be because of the infant's immaturity and vulnerability. Longer stretches of sleep are associated with increased risk of sudden infant death syndrome (SIDS), so frequent waking is protective (Schechtman *et al.* 1992). Babies should not be forced into longer stretches of sleep, but some do spontaneously fall into this pattern at around three months, and that seems to be fine.

Of course babies feed for all sorts of reasons, not just hunger and thirst. They may feed because they are too hot or too cold – the skin contact helps them regulate their body temperature. They may feed because they are in pain, as breastfeeding gives pain relief to a baby. They may feed because they are lonely and scared. Babies who find themselves alone are hardwired to call out, as they think they have fallen off their mother, which goes back to the times where we had fur and our babies clung. They will need a feed to recover from the trauma of finding themselves in the cot. They may feed because they are bored, we all do this! They may feed because they are feeling unwell – our milk is full of antibodies to help them recover, and we make antibodies to any specific virus baby may have come into contact with. Breastfed babies still get ill, but they often are less severely ill and recover quickly. They may feed because they are growing their bodies or their brains. They may feed because they are tired and want to go to sleep easily, and there is absolutely no harm in doing this. Lots of baby books say it is a bad habit – it is not, it is biologically normal.

Adding all of these factors together, the majority of breastfed babies like to feed every one and a half to three hours, not evenly spaced, and with some periods of frequent feeding. So parents need to understand that they will be spending a lot of time feeding in the early days. As they get older babies sometimes stretch out a little, and they also become more efficient and so the feeds become shorter. Tandem feeding (feeding both babies at the same time on a breast each) can maximise the gap between feeds.

Babies do not feed at set intervals of time, and the gaps between feeds vary depending on all sorts of factors. For example, cluster feeding is a normal newborn behaviour. Cluster feeding is a term that means babies need to go back on the breast several times in a row before they will settle, and cluster feeding periods usually tie in with the times of day where babies are often naturally more alert or fussy, as well as in the early hours of the morning. Parents often feel like there cannot be any more available milk, but production is going on in the background all the time and breasts are actually never empty, so each time the baby is latched on they will trigger another milk ejection reflex. Full term babies often cluster feed at night in the very early days and then it moves to the evening period from around three weeks up until three months or so, although some continue longer – and the timings can be a bit different for early babies. Learning how to tandem feed helps massively during these times as the parent can feed and calm both babies simultaneously.

Babies may develop a pattern where they have one or two longer stretches of sleep in each 24-hour period. Often this is after the evening cluster feed, so it is a good plan for the parents to go to bed as well and make the most of it. Babies also often sleep well during the first nap in the morning, so this can be a good time for parents to stay in bed and get an extra hour of sleep, or to get up and have a shower and get ready for the day if that is something that is important to them. As long as the babies are generally alert and waking themselves for feeds, and weight gain and nappy output is good, it is fine to leave the babies to sleep for a bit longer if it is led by them.

Babies do not like to be put down very much in the early days. This period is commonly known as the fourth trimester. As humans we birth our babies quite early in their gestation, and newborn human babies are consequently very immature. In order to keep safe and warm our babies prefer to settle and sleep on their mother's chest, but sometimes a partner or family member will do. They need to feel comfort, security, warmth, and to be close to their source of food. Babies cannot be spoiled with too much cuddling, and responding to their needs as much as possible helps to build the secure attachment that is so important in their first 1001 days.

Humans are 'carry' mammals, as are all the apes and also marsupials. 'Carry' mammals birth the most immature infants – much more immature than other mammals. They are completely dependent on their mothers for food, warmth, and safety. In addition human babies are born far earlier in their development than all other primates because of the combination of our large brains (making our heads large) and our upright walking (which makes our hips narrow). This means human babies are quite helpless and vulnerable at birth. Only marsupials, of all mammals, birth their babies at an earlier stage in their gestation. Kangaroo babies are born very premature, but manage to crawl up into the mother's pouch and continue their gestation, latching onto the mother's nipple and feeding fairly continuously.

Trying to replicate this close contact with our human babies is beneficial. The human baby's habitat is the breastfeeding parent's chest. A sling can be used to replicate the pouch and means the parent can give the babies the closeness they need while still having hands free to do other things if necessary.

'Carry' mammals have milk that is high in lactose for brain growth and lower in protein and fat as our babies feed frequently. Other types of mammal are 'follow', 'nest', and 'cache' mammals. 'Follow' mammals, such as horses and giraffes, can walk soon after birth and they feed quite frequently as they can keep up with their mothers. Their milk is a little higher in fat and protein than 'carry' mammals as they feed a little less frequently, and need to build muscle and strength to walk long distances from a very young age. 'Nest' mammals such as dogs and cats leave their babies and return to feed every four to six hours, which means that their milk needs to be higher in fat and protein to help them wait for their parents return. Finally, there are 'cache' animals such as rabbits and deer. They leave their babies in a safe place and return every 12 hours or so to feed them. Consequently, their milk is much higher in fat and protein in order to sustain them for long periods.

Many of our baby books seem to think humans are 'nest' mammals and our babies should feed only every four hours and be put in their cot to sleep in between. But this just is not how we have evolved. Human babies expect to be held constantly and fed frequently. Our milk is the perfect consistency for this. This is normal newborn human behaviour.

Find a support system

As we have learned so far, having a new baby is a time consuming and intense affair. Add into the mix the fact there are two or three babies, and accessing some support can be incredibly beneficial.

Partners and/or close family can be a big support. It is helpful if they can do some research into breastfeeding and normal newborn behaviour, so they are more able to help and understand what is usual – maybe they could accompany the parents to an antenatal breastfeeding session or watch one online. There has been a lot of research into baby behaviour since the previous generation was raising their babies and a lot of guidelines have changed. A spare pair of hands or two can really help with the amount of cuddles needed! Some cultures have a 40-day post-partum period where the family looks after the mother and helps with the baby. Whether a formal timescale is something they feel they would like to do or not, it is essential in these early weeks to slow down and focus on getting to know new babies, establishing breastfeeding, and recovering from pregnancy and birth.

In the UK their community midwife, followed by their health visitor, will be a parent's first port of call for support in the early days. In other countries it is the paediatrician or family nurse who will be there for concerns. But these health care professionals often only have very basic knowledge of infant feeding, so more specialist breastfeeding support may sometimes be necessary. It can be good for parents to find out what is available in their local area before the babies arrive, so they are prepared. They can find out if there is a local breastfeeding support group, Breastfeeding Counsellor or International Board Certified Lactation Consultant (IBCLC). It can be a good plan to pop into a local breastfeeding group before the babies arrive just to see how it works, and maybe make contact with a Breastfeeding Counsellor or IBCLC so the parents know how they work and how to get hold of them if needed.

Antenatal hand expressing colostrum

Twins are generally born a bit small, a bit sleepy and a bit more difficult to feed, so they often need a little bit of extra colostrum in the early days. Parents can be supported to hand express alongside breastfeeding once the babies have arrived, but it can be good to have a head start by collecting some in the latter weeks or days of pregnancy. Antenatal hand expressing was found to improve maternal confidence in breastfeeding (Brisbane & Giglia 2013).

Antenatal hand expressing has been proven to be safe from 36 weeks of pregnancy (Forster *et al.* 2017). However, as many twins are born at or around 36 weeks, if a birth is planned for around this time then parents can have a discussion with their health care professionals to assess their particular risk factors and work out a plan. For example, it can work well to start in the week leading up to a planned induction or caesarean section. Some can also be harvested once the parent is in labour or in the run up to their caesarean section if they are at higher risk.

We usually suggest hand expressing rather than pumping as it is gentler, and colostrum is so thick and sticky and in such small quantities that it would just get lost in a breast pump. It is totally normal to only get very small amounts – colostrum is concentrated, packed full of immunity, and all that baby needs in the first few days, so every drop counts.

We usually suggest trying hand expressing two or three times a day. The colostrum can be collected in syringes, either straight from the nipple, or into a sterilised cup first and then transferred to a syringe. Parents can add to the same syringe over the course of the day if the amounts are small. All the syringes should be labelled clearly with the parent's name, date, and hospital number, and then they can be frozen in a lidded container or freezer bag to avoid any contamination. When it is time to have the babies, take syringes to the hospital in a cool bag, and make sure the staff know. Some hospitals will be able to keep it in the freezer, others will only have a fridge available. If only a fridge is available and there is an induction, it may be worth waiting until established labour has begun, as colostrum has to be used within 24 hours of fully defrosting. If the parent has collected a large amount of colostrum, leaving some at home is a good idea in case of mistakes, and the partner can always pick up more from home if needed. There is more information on hand expressing technique later in the book.

What do multiple birth parents need to breastfeed?
Of course, parents only actually need babies and breasts to breastfeed. If the babies are feeding well, no specialist equipment is necessary. However, there are a few things that some parents find helpful.

Twin breastfeeding pillow?
There are several tandem feeding positions which can be done without pillows or cushions at all. However, if the parents would like to tandem feed, a good supportive breastfeeding pillow can help to support the babies at the correct height. It is important to take into account the body shape of the parent when choosing a cushion as not all pillows on the market suit everyone – those that are shorter with

larger breasts will need a lower pillow than those that are taller with smaller breasts. Some may prefer to just use household cushions and pillows, or a pregnancy pillow. Many do a laid back position as their first tandem feed after birth which does not need a feeding pillow, and if staying in the hospital it can be a bit difficult to tandem feed due to narrow beds and unsuitable chairs, so leaving a pillow in the car in case is probably a good plan.

At home, parents often find they need to have a different set up for the bed than they do for the sofa, generally because we tend to lean back more with our legs out in front of us on the bed. Sometimes breastfeeding pillows may need tweaking a bit with the addition of cushions under the front or sides if the pillow is too low, or under the parent if it is too high. When I do a breastfeeding consultation in the home with a twin family who want to learn to tandem feed, we generally collect up every cushion and pillow in the house and experiment!

Breast pump?

It is true that many multiple birth families do pump a bit, either through necessity or because they wish to. However, I generally suggest to hold off buying one until the babies have arrived, as different pumps are suitable for different scenarios. If the babies are born early, in the neonatal unit, not latching, or latching but not feeding efficiently, it is best to use a hospital grade double pump or multi-user pump. Hospitals have these pumps available while the parents are in, and once they are discharged home they can borrow, hire, or buy one for home use. It is important to use a hospital grade double pump as they are the most efficient at removing the milk, robust enough to be used frequently and thus the parent tends to get a greater yield. If the babies are full term and feeding well it is actually better to wait a few weeks before introducing bottles and pumping, as it can interfere with establishing milk production and babies can be more prone to bottle preference.

If the parent decides to pump occasionally at this stage, a cheaper double electric pump will be the fastest, but a single electric pump, hand pump, silicone pump, or even just hand expressing can be just as effective. Bear in mind some single electric occasional pumps are just as expensive as some of the hospital grade double pumps, so shop wisely!

Bottles?

Many parents may need to use a bottle for top ups in the early weeks, or perhaps just for convenience later on. Bottles are not items that need to be bought in advance, as until the babies arrive it will not be clear if they are necessary. Ideally if breastfeeding is going well it is a good plan to leave introducing a bottle until a few weeks down the line. However, if the babies are not feeding effectively, it may be necessary to supplement in the first few weeks and bottles are often chosen for this purpose. Bottles are by no means the only way of supplementing though – there are a number of other options: syringe, finger feeding, cup, spoon, supplementary nursing system.

Generally, it is much better to go for a medium neck bottle with a gentle slope on the teat. Baby will be able to get a deeper latch onto the bottle and the teat will go up deep into the roof of the mouth. Not only will this help bottle feeding, but it will also help the babies continue to latch onto the breast. The bottles that profess to be breast-shaped do not actually resemble a breast in a baby's mouth. A breast is drawn into the baby's mouth and compressed. A bottle with a wide neck shape does not compress and means that baby cannot get a deep latch and will just feed from the end of the teat. This shallow latch is something we most definitely want to avoid when breastfeeding.

Formula?

Many people will tell parents they will need formula 'just in case'. If you choose to formula feed, in United Nations Children's Fund (UNICEF) baby friendly accredited hospitals you will need to provide your own. But if you wish to breastfeed and there is a clinical need for infant formula, the hospital will provide it. Instead of 'just in case' formula, why not take some harvested colostrum instead? Once home, in societies where we have 24-hour supermarkets, there is no need to get any formula in advance unless you plan to use it from birth. It can be very tempting during those epic early cluster feeding sessions to turn to it if it is in the cupboard, but if the goal is to exclusively breastfeed then using formula will not help long term. Having said that, some people do find comfort in having some in the cupboard.

Bedside cot?

Not directly related to breastfeeding, but a large bedside cot, either shop bought or adapted from a standard cot, really does make responding to the babies at night much easier. The babies can share a sleep space and research has shown they may get some comfort from each other. They can either sleep horizontally across the cot or at one end next to each other to begin with. Being able to put the babies down without having to get out of bed and lower them into a standard cot helps settle them more easily, and you can respond to them waking for night feeds quickly without even having to get out of bed. Safer sleep guidelines suggest to position babies on their backs to sleep (also called supine) on a firm flat surface, with feet to the edge of the cot to prevent them from slipping down under the blankets if they wriggle.

Sling?

Again not directly related to feeding, a sling can be a big help in the early days. Babies really do not like to be put down in the first few months. They often spend lots of time sleeping on the feeding cushion between feeds in contact with the parent, or perhaps with one baby on each parent's chest. But if parents need to get things done, a sling can give the babies the closeness and comfort they need while allowing the wearer the use of their hands. A stretchy wrap type sling can be used for one or both babies in the early days, and there are a host of single and twin carriers on the market. Finding a local sling consultant to do a tutorial can be helpful to ensure babies are being positioned safely in the sling or carrier. And it is possible to breastfeed in a sling, even tandem breastfeed!

What can partners do?

Often partners are worried that they will not have much to do if the babies are breastfed. But with two or three babies there is plenty to do and plenty of opportunities to bond.

- Look after siblings – older children often need lots of support with the adjustment to new babies in the house. For the breastfeeding parent it is really important for them to have the time and support to establish breastfeeding in the early weeks. Doing this with a toddler or pre-schooler in tow is challenging, so someone to give them attention is invaluable.

- Take charge of bedtime with the older children – babies are often very unsettled in the evenings and like to cluster feed for hours, which can make bedtimes with older children very difficult.

- Take over the housework – the housework will always be there, unfortunately, and this is something that just cannot be achieved when looking after multiple new babies. If the partner cannot manage it, consider a cleaner if you can afford to pay, or a rota of friends and family.

- Provide snacks, drinks, and meals – breastfeeding is hungry and thirsty work. The saying goes 'Feed the mother so the mother can feed the baby.' This is very true, and cooking is very difficult with new babies. Parents can rope in friends and family to fill the freezer with nutritious food and drop meals on the doorstep. When the partner returns to work, leaving the breastfeeding parent a packed lunch in the fridge which they can just grab when they have a chance is very helpful. Sometimes in the chaos it is easy to forget to eat.

- Make sure the breastfeeding parent has everything they need – there is nothing worse than being stuck feeding babies with rubbish on the TV and the remote across the other side of the room. They can also find the phone charger!

- Change babies – what goes in one end comes out of the other. Babies need changing a lot. They should be doing at least six wet nappies and a couple of poos every day. Multiply this by two or three babies and that's a lot of nappy changes!

- Pass babies for feeding – in the early days having some help to pass and position babies is invaluable. It takes a lot of practice to be able to set up to feed, and babies seem so small and fragile to begin with, so the extra pair of hands makes a big difference.

- Settle babies – partners are often better at settling babies after a feed than the breastfeeding parent. They do not smell of milk, which can make the new baby less confused about whether it's feeding time or not! Cuddling, and doing some skin to skin, is lovely. It is very beneficial to the babies and also strengthens the parent's bond with the baby. Rocking, patting, and tiger in the tree position are great ways to settle a fussy baby. (Tiger in the tree position is where baby lies on their tummy along the parent's forearm, head supported by the bend in the elbow.) Wearing babies in a sling, bathing and massaging them are all ways partners can bond.

- Top up feeds – if babies need some top ups, the breastfeed–express–top up 'triple feeding' routine is very intense. Partners can do the top up feeds while the breastfeeding parent pumps, which makes feeding a little more efficient. Some families also make the decision to do one bottle feed of expressed breast milk (or formula) a day to let the nursing parent get some sleep.

- Take babies out for a walk every day – taking them out for half an hour can give the breastfeeding parent a break. They can choose to sleep, have a bath or shower, or just sit and not be touched for a few minutes. Babies will often settle when moving so it can work well.

- Take the babies in the morning – the partner can get up with the babies after the first feed so the breastfeeding parent can stay in bed and get some extra sleep, or take a shower. Babies are often quite settled in the mornings.

- Be a gatekeeper, managing visitors – it can be very over-whelming in the early days when everybody wants to see the new arrivals. Partners are vital to plan these visits and keep them manageable. When establishing breastfeeding it can be very stressful if family stay for long periods, especially if the nursing parent is not comfortable to feed in front of them. Visitors must understand that to earn a cuddle they must do something useful and not expect to be waited on!

- Encourage breastfeeding, learn about breastfeeding, defend the decision to breastfeed – learning about all the benefits of breastfeeding, keeping the breastfeeding parent motivated in the difficult times and celebrating each small achievement is a vital role of a supportive partner. Some friends and family members may not understand the decision to breastfeed, especially if they did not breastfeed themselves, which can lead to comments which are not necessarily supportive. Often these come from a place of love and concern, but it can get very wearing always having to defend the decision or resist offers to give a bottle.

- Find breastfeeding support – if breastfeeding is not going well then accessing breastfeeding support is vital. Partners can take the lead in finding this support. They can search for their local breastfeeding support group, infant feeding team or IBCLC, and make an appointment.

Visitors – here are the rules!

- Visitors should make sure they phone/text first. They should not just turn up – it may not be a good time.

- Bring food – cooking is really difficult with new babies and new parents need nutritious food to help have enough energy to look after them. If visitors cannot bring food they could order takeaway or give frozen meals from a delivery service.

- Make the tea – visitors should not expect to be waited on. They should put the kettle on and make tea for themselves and the new parents. And bring cake!

- Do some chores – while they are waiting for the kettle to boil, maybe empty the dishwasher, wipe down the surfaces, hang up the laundry, or ask if any jobs need doing.

- Wash hands – new babies have underdeveloped immune systems. The last thing new parents want is sick babies.

- Stay home if they are ill – new babies may be quite poorly even with just mild viruses. Plus new parents really do not need to get ill! They have enough to deal with. Visitors should be prepared to wait a bit; babies are babies for many months and there will be other chances.

- No kissing babies – the herpes simplex virus, which causes cold sores, can be deadly to a baby.

- No unsolicited advice – of course visitors can ask how the parents are doing, that is just polite. And if the parents ask their opinion on something then it is fine to share experiences, but they must be sure that the parents realise this is just their own experience, and it may not apply to every parent/baby.

- Be careful not to outstay their welcome – new babies can get overstimulated with lots of people around and new parents can feel overwhelmed and overtired with lots of visitors. Stay for a short time, help out, have a quick cuddle if it is appropriate, and then leave.

- Parents may still need help and support when the baby is a bit older. Often the offers dry up after the first few weeks, so see if they need help with anything later on.

Top Tips for Parents

Take time to process the news.

Tell people there's more than one when you are ready.

Acknowledge your feelings and worries.

Try to break it down into specific worries – this makes things seem less daunting.

Ask questions at antenatal appointments, write a list to take with you as you think of them.

Ask for evidence of any suggestion if it does not line up with your understanding.

Remember it is your choice how you birth your babies. Health care professionals can offer suggestions and should be able to back these up with research. Risks and benefits of every decision should always be discussed.

If you do not understand any health concerns ask if your health care professional can provide you with some further information.

Learn about pregnancy, birth, breastfeeding, and babies! Educate yourself.

Find a multiple birth antenatal session if there is one, online ones are also available.

Find an antenatal breastfeeding session, online ones are also available.

Join online communities.

Find your local support network: breastfeeding support and post-natal support.

Plan for family and friends to help out – even if it is just a neighbour leaving a meal on your doorstep.

If you have older children, make plans for when you are having the babies, but also for the first few weeks after the babies are born. Help with the school run, play dates, mealtimes, bedtime, toddler entertainment are all worth considering.

If you have a budget, find paid support. Ask for donations towards a doula, cleaner, or IBCLC as new baby presents from friends and relations. Consider childcare options for older children.

Do as much research into feeding as you do into birth or which pram to buy.

If you are at risk of premature delivery, ask to look around the neonatal unit.

Ask your health care professionals about antenatal hand expressing if you need to start before 36 weeks gestation.

Discuss with friends and family about your decision to breast-feed and how you wish to be supported.

— Chapter 3 —

Premature Bi _

According to the charity Twins Trust, around 40% of UK twins need some extra support after birth and go to the neonatal unit (NNU) or special care baby unit (SCBU) (Twins Trust 2021). If the babies need more intensive care they may go to the neonatal intensive care unit (NICU). This can be a very worrying time for parents. If there is any warning that the babies may arrive early, parents can go and look around the neonatal unit so they know what to expect. It can be quite a daunting place full of wires and beeps. Being shown around in advance, and having the different parts explained, can take away some of the worry.

It can be a good idea to try collecting some colostrum before the babies arrive. This can act as insurance against the babies needing a boost in the first hours, as well as providing expressing practice which is a handy skill to learn. If the babies will be born earlier than 36 weeks gestation parents will need to talk this through with their health care practitioners to discuss the risks versus benefits of ante-natal expressing. As discussed in the section on antenatal expressing in Chapter 2, research has shown that it is safe from 36 weeks (Forster *et al.* 2017), but there is no research regarding the risks of collecting colostrum before 36 weeks. Some hospitals are now encouraging antenatal hand expressing during active labour of a preterm birth or in the six hours leading up to a scheduled caesarean section. It is worth discussing this with health care providers as even a tiny amount can make a difference to the babies.

Parents could ask about having a delivery room cuddle. Many premature babies are actually quite stable straight after birth and as concluded that, with appropriate safeguards, delivery cuddles are feasible and achievable even for extremely preterm babies, irrespective of birth gestation. Facilitation of the cuddle is an early and very important family-centred care practice, which seems much appreciated by parents and which may improve bonding, lactation, and maternal mental health (Clarke *et al.* 2021). If the babies are very early or unwell, this could be the only time the parents get to hold the babies for many days or weeks. It is a very precious moment in a very stressful situation and can help encourage shocked parents to accept the situation, feel like the babies belong to them, and be more involved in their care.

The composition of preterm milk is different to the milk of full term babies. The book *Breastfeeding and Human Lactation* states:

> The milk of a woman who delivers a preterm infant is different from that of a woman who delivers at term, probably to meet the needs of the low-birth-weight neonate. Compared with term human milk, preterm human milk has higher levels of energy, lipids, protein, nitrogen, fatty acids, some vitamins and immune factors. In addition, preterm milk has higher levels of immune factors, including cells, immunoglobulins, and anti-inflammatory elements, than term human milk. (Wambach & Spencer 2021, p.107)

It is highly valued in the neonatal unit and parents are generally supported to hand express colostrum preferably within the first six hours after birth. Following on from this, hand expressing frequently should be encouraged. Once milk volumes begin to increase parents can move onto the pump to provide breast milk for tube feeds. The hospital should be able to advise on renting a hospital grade double pump for when the lactating parent is discharged. It is gently recommended to pump 8–12 times in 24 hours making sure at least one is between 2 and 5am when hormone levels are at their highest.

Hand expressing

Once the babies are born it is important to begin hand expressing within the first couple of hours after birth if possible. Parents should ask for support with this, but knowing the theory before babies arrive can help, especially if staff are busy.

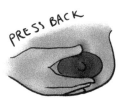 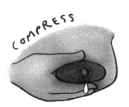 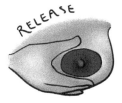

To start they should gently massage the whole breast and the nipple for a couple of minutes. This stimulates the oxytocin and helps move the colostrum down into the breast making it easier to extract. Place fingers and thumb around the breast in a C shape about an inch or 2–2.5cm back from the nipple. The parent should be able to feel the ducts. Everyone has their own 'sweet spot' where the colostrum begins to come more easily, so they will need to experiment a bit, and do lots of practice! Push back into the chest wall, then squeeze fingers and thumb together and hold for a couple of seconds. Repeat. They should start to get a drop or two after a few goes, although some-times it takes quite a long time to come. Sometimes the colostrum can look quite transparent to start with, and then the thick sticky golden liquid comes through – although colostrum does vary, and some people find it is always a paler colour. Sliding fingers down the breast should be avoided as is not very effective, and will make the skin sore. A slow firm squeeze and hold is more effective than a fast light squeeze. They should move their hands around the areola to ensure they stimulate all the ducts and swap hands and breasts once the first one slows down or their hand gets tired. Midwives are often very experienced in the technique of hand expressing and can provide good support for parents to learn what to do.

Colostrum tends to be stored in syringes as then it can be given direct to the baby, put into the feeding tube, used for oral care, or stored easily. Colostrum can either be sucked into a syringe straight from the nipple if is in small drops, or collected in a small cup and then sucked up into the syringe.

It is good idea to hand express every two to three hours to mimic what the baby would be doing if they were feeding directly. This will help prime the prolactin receptors in the breast and encourage future milk production (Hill *et al.* 2005). A pump can also be used for added stimulation, but the thick sticky colostrum is in such small quantities that it tends to get lost in the pump, so hand expressing is often more effective for the actual collection. Babies only need a small quantity of colostrum, so every drop counts. It is so concentrated and full of antibodies that it is like giving babies their first vaccination.

Many people who have supported parents through hand expressing for a premature baby or non-latching baby may have noticed that after the initial few hand expressing sessions, the volume of expressed colostrum often decreases. A recent study has found parents can express a greater volume of expressed milk in the first 12 hours post-partum, than in the next 18 hours. By 30 hours post-partum, the volume of colostrum begins to increase exponentially as secretary activation occurs, commonly known as milk 'coming in'. This decline in expressed milk volume during the early post-partum period often causes concern among parents. Therefore, information around this normal trajectory of human milk volume should be shared (Kato *et al.* 2022).

Pumping to establish milk production

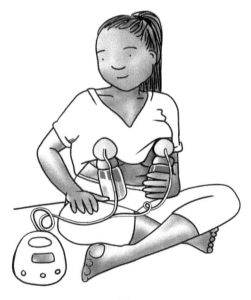

Milk begins to 'come in' around day 2–5 after birth, a process called 'Lactogenesis ll'. This process is triggered by the birth of the placenta and will happen whether the birthing parent is breastfeeding, pumping or doing neither. The colostrum gradually changes into transitional milk and becomes more watery in consistency, and the quantities become larger. This is a good time to introduce the pump. Over the course of the first week or so transitional milk will change into mature milk, which is lighter in colour and available in larger volumes.

Hospital grade pumps should be available to use in hospital. Maternity departments often have a pumping room, and they may also be able to facilitate pumping by the side of the babies' incubator.

To establish a full supply via expressing can be challenging. Pumps, although very effective, are just not as efficient as a full term baby who is feeding well, with all the hormonal stimulation this provides. Here are some tips to help establish milk production when pumping.

Frequency

There really is no better way to get a full supply than to pump frequently; 8 to 10 times a day is ideal to begin with. Some parents with larger storage capacities may be able to drop a couple of sessions and continue to make enough milk for their babies but, for many, frequency is the key to establishing and maintaining a good supply of milk. These expressing sessions do not need to be evenly spaced, but it is not advisable to leave it longer than three to four hours between pumping sessions. Pumping during the night is particularly important as it is well known that levels of prolactin, the milk making hormone, are higher at night. If milk is not removed during this time it may have an impact on the amount of milk it is possible to express. If the parent misses a pumping session for some reason, it is better to shuffle up the others so they still achieve the same number over 24 hours. Parents may find that around 15–20 minutes of pumping is sufficient. However, if the milk is still flowing it would be good to continue. Some parents find they will not get much more after the first 10 minutes – it is very individual. So it is really important for them to get to know what works best for their body and their situation. One study found:

Of the four main milk ejection patterns identified, each removed a similar percentage of the available milk but varied in the time to reach 80% of the total expression volume. The first two milk ejections produced the greatest percentage (62%) of total milk volume during breast expression. (Prime *et al.* 2011, pp.183–190)

So we can conclude that in general many will find shorter pumping sessions more frequently are more effective at establishing a good supply than longer sessions less frequently.

Efficiency

Using a hospital grade multi-user pump is recommended. Not only are these pumps more efficient but they are robust and will manage frequent use. In hospital the staff should be able to provide one for parents to use. These are normally available in the pumping room; sometimes by baby's cot or incubator. Once discharged, hospital grade pumps can sometimes be borrowed from the hospital or the community, or be hired either direct from the manufacturer, online, or from a local pump agent. Sometimes the hospital may have a discount code arrangement with one of the manufacturers. There are a couple of cheaper hospital grade pumps that can be bought and used long term.

Breast shell size

It is essential that the sizing of the pump's breast shell is correct for the nursing parent's anatomy. This will ensure pumping is comfortable and will also help maximise milk production. A pair of breasts are not identical, so may need two shells of different sizes. Sometimes the parent may need to change size as they go through their pumping journey, as breast and nipple sizes change. Nipple diameter is the key – if the areola is drawn into the shaft this means the shell is too big. If the nipple is rubbing on the sides of the shaft this means the shaft is too small. Check the manufacturer's information for what sizes are available and how to check yours is correct.

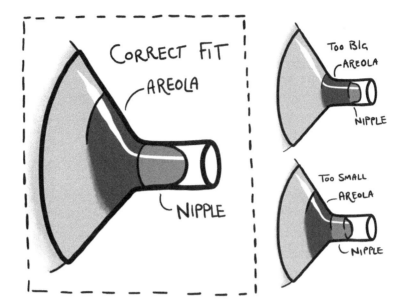

Double pumping

As well as being less time consuming because both breasts can be pumped at the same time, research shows parents make more milk (Fewtrell *et al.* 2016) and can increase milk ejections and calorie content of the milk (Prime *et al.* 2012).

Hands-on pumping technique

A technique which incorporates gentle massage, hand expressing, and pumping all at the same time. Many have found that this can greatly increase output and one study found it increased yield by 48% (Morton *et al.* 2009). A further study found that this technique increased calorie and fat content of the milk (Morton *et al.* 2012). The parent massages the breast and the nipple for a couple of minutes before the pumping session to stimulate the flow of oxytocin and help the milk be more easily available. The parent continues to massage and hand express while pumping. After the flow has slowed, finishing with some further hand expressing can get a little more milk. In order to do this effectively while double pumping, a hands free pumping bra will be needed.

A hands free pumping bra can make the above massage much easier, as the bra is used to hold the cones of the pump in place and so hands are free. It also means that parents can pump and do other things at the same time. This can be essential, especially with older children. Hands free pumping bras can be bought, or made by cutting holes in an old bra or crop top in line with the nipples. The cones are inserted through the holes.

Power (or cluster) pumping

The idea behind power pumping is that it mimics a baby's natural cluster feeding pattern and this can help stimulate milk production. It has also been found that the initial milk ejection reflex yields as much as 45% of the available milk (Ramsay *et al.* 2006). Stimulating a new milk ejection reflex after a gap could potentially increase the total yield, rather than experiencing a second or third ejection during a longer pumping session. Each time the milk ejection reflex is stimulated, there will be a spike in prolactin, the milk making hormone, which may lead to more milk in the future. The following is a pattern regularly suggested to parents for double and single pumping. It can be done once a day.

Power pumping

Double pump	Single pump
Pump 20 mins	Pump left 10 mins
Rest 10 mins	Pump right 10 mins
Pump 10 mins	Rest 5 mins
Rest 10 mins	Pump left 10 mins
Pump 10 mins	Pump right 10 mins
	Rest 5 mins
	Pump left 10 mins
	Pump right 10 mins

Another, less strict, variant of power pumping or cluster pumping is to set up the pump for a couple of hours somewhere in the house that is passed frequently. Every time the parent walks past, they pump for five minutes.

Warmth

Applying a warm compress just before the expressing session can help stimulate the let-down reflex and encourage the milk to flow.

Skin to skin with baby

Skin to skin, for example during kangaroo care, helps boost oxytocin and encourages the milk to flow. Oxytocin is one of the key hormones involved in the delivery of milk stimulating the milk ejection reflex, or let-down reflex, meaning milk flows more easily when pumping.

Look at baby

Look at photos, videos, pictures, pumping next to the cot, listening to your baby, with clothes or fabric that smell of your baby. All these remind the breasts what they are supposed to be doing! They also stimulate oxytocin and help with bonding and milk production.

Latch baby

If baby is beginning to latch on to the breast, pumping straight afterwards can encourage the milk to flow, as the baby will have stimulated the let-down reflex. The stimulus of a baby suckling at the breast is different to that of a pump and may increase supply.

Distraction

'A watched pot never boils.' It's the same with pumping. If you watch what you get, you are likely to get less milk. Distraction with music, relaxation recordings, mindfulness, watching TV programmes (preferably happy, entertaining ones), chatting to other mums or friends and family have all been found to increase milk production. Stress can inhibit the milk ejection reflex as the stress hormone cortisol travels down the same pathways as oxytocin, so these relaxation and distraction techniques can help keep the milk flowing.

Eat and drink specific foods

Of course eating a healthy balanced diet is good for the health and energy of the parent, but there is no evidence that diet affects milk production by itself, despite what is often said. It is important that the breastfeeding parent eats to their hunger and drinks to their thirst, as getting enough is important, but there is no evidence that any specific foodstuffs make a difference to supply in themselves.

Galactagogues

There are many herbs or medications out there which either have some scientific evidence behind them or have anecdotal evidence that they can help to increase milk production. However, none of these work unless the milk is being removed frequently from the breast. They are not a magic wand. Please make sure when finding information that you look for a reputable, unbiased source. The book *Making More Milk: The Breastfeeding Guide to Increasing Your Milk Production* (Marasco & West 2019) has a very comprehensive chapter on galactagogues and the most recent research.

Rest

It is really key for parents to rest. Of course it is essential to wake in the night to pump in order to get a good supply, but getting a good amount of sleep is so vital to cope with the stresses and strains that the neonatal unit involves. Get help with all the usual household chores, looking after older children, and cooking. Feeling relaxed will help the milk flow.

It is important to look at 24-hour output, not necessarily what is expressed in each session. This is because there is often a wide variation in amounts from different times of day, and almost all mothers make more milk in one breast in comparison to the other. Over the first few weeks we hope to see a gradual increase in volume in each 24-hour period.

PERSONAL STORY
Hannah with Josh and Tommy

My boys were tube fed in the NICU, which meant my breast-feeding journey started with me pumping. For the first 24 hours or so they were too poorly for any milk at all, and instead were on a glucose drip. This gave me the chance to get a slight head start on building my supply. Then from day 2 they started being fed tiny amounts of my milk – initially I hand expressed just a ml or so at a time, then progressed onto pumping using the hospital grade pump. Once we knew I would be leaving the hospital while the boys were still there we ordered a hospital grade double pump to use at home. I followed the advice of pumping 8–10 times in every 24 hours. I had a notebook and enjoyed ticking off each session – it gave me a focus and made me feel as though I was doing something useful. Pumping can be hard work, and it can be so frustrating when you only get a tiny amount from a pumping session. I always found I got more if I had just had a nap. When we left the hospital, in addition to the two boys in car seats, we had a great big cold bag of frozen breast milk to come home with us, which lasted us for the occasional bottle for many months to come!

Top Tips for Parents in the Neonatal Unit

As discussed in the previous section, parents should make sure, once they are discharged, that they have access to a hospital grade double pump if possible.

Parents should be encouraged to ask questions and make sure they are consulted on everything. If they do not understand something, they should be encouraged to ask what it means. Writing down questions as they think of them will help them to remember when the doctor comes round, and writing notes about what the doctors say will help them to remember later, especially if trying to relay information back to their partner or family members.

Parents should be encouraged to be fully involved in their babies' care. Parents often comment that it does not feel like the babies belong to them as they are being looked after by the nurses and doctors, but there are plenty of things they can do. Learning how to look after the babies under the guidance of the nurses will help parents to gain confidence for when they are discharged home.

Establishing breastfeeding with premature babies can be quite challenging and takes a lot of patience. It is really helpful if the parents can find the most supportive and informed staff. If there is an infant feeding lead they will be able to talk them through the different steps in order to establish direct breastfeeding.

Ensure that the staff talk through the risks and benefits of giving formula or fortifier. Parents should be fully informed before making a decision to supplement. Donor milk may be an option if the babies do need to be supplemented – hospitals often have certain criteria that a baby will need to meet, but it is always worth asking. Parents do not have to introduce bottles to get home more quickly, although they may find that the babies will continue to need to be topped up for a little while once they are discharged. Sometimes babies can be sent home still having some of their feeds through a tube, or using a cup or bottle.

At home it is very helpful for parents to have a support network around them to provide food and look after the adults while they spend time with the babies, especially if there are older children to think of. These supporters can fill the freezer with nutritious food, run the vacuum round, give lifts to the hospital and do the school run.

Finding other families in the same situation can really help people to cope with the hospital environment. Parents should be encouraged to get chatting to others in the pumping room, and to investigate support groups they can join locally, online, and on social media.

Self-care is incredibly important. Parents need to make sure they eat, drink, and sleep. It is ok for them to have a break and do something for themselves while the babies are being looked after by very capable hospital staff. It is ok to leave.

Taking pictures of everything, even the painful bits, will give them something to look back on some day. It is so important to celebrate every milestone, no matter how small. Celebrate every drop of breast milk provided – every drop makes a difference.

Transitioning premature babies onto the breast

Efficient rooting, areolar grasp, and latching on have been observed as early as 28 weeks gestation, while nutritive sucking has been observed from just before 31 weeks gestation, and longer sucking bursts from 32 weeks (Nyqvist, Sjödén & Ewald 1999). So once the babies are stable and rooting is observed they can be offered the breast during kangaroo care.

Learning to breastfeed as a premature baby is a long, slow, tiring process and it requires everybody to have lots of patience. To start with babies can have skin to skin time, or kangaroo care, be encouraged to explore the nipple, and possibly have a few sucks. A baby can begin with non-nutritive sucking at a recently pumped breast to provide a gentle experience without an overwhelming flow of milk. Once they are used to this, a fuller breast can be introduced, but at this early stage the majority of any feed will still be expressed milk through the feeding tube. The staff will encourage parents to try baby at the breast once or twice a day, so as not to tire them out. Once they become stronger and start to suck and swallow more efficiently they can move on to more frequent feeds. Tube feeds can be given at the breast so the babies begin to associate the act of breastfeeding with the feeling of satiety.

A nipple shield can help the smaller baby to latch onto the breast, especially if they have been given bottles. There is evidence that suggests shields can significantly increase milk intake in preterm infants (Meier *et al.* 2000). Introducing a nipple shield is of course another intervention – when making the decision, it is important to consider how the lactating parent is responding to pumping. If a parent is finding pumping is working well then it may be appropriate to wait for the babies to become more effective direct on the breast, and not introduce the nipple shield. However, if the parent is struggling with achieving a good yield from pumping, introducing the shield can encourage the babies to breastfeed more effectively more quickly, and this will help with milk production. The majority of babies will be able to breastfeed effectively without the use of a shield as they reach full term.

Babies will gradually be able to move towards exclusive breastfeeding as they become stronger and more coordinated. This can be at different ages for different babies – including different multiple babies from the same family. For some it can be around the 36–37 week gestation mark, while others need to get to nearer or even after full term. Some babies will be able to move straight on to exclusive breastfeeding from tube feeding, although this new enthusiasm for feeding can be a bit misleading as the suck can still be uncoordinated and inefficient, and the babies can still tire easily. If we move on to exclusive breastfeeding too quickly it can cause problems with babies not taking enough milk and becoming too tired, and then their weight gain may slow. For some babies it is advisable to continue to top up with expressed breast milk for a few weeks while the babies continue to increase their muscle tone and coordination. Many parents will choose to remove tubes and supplement using a different method so the babies can go home more quickly, however babies can be discharged tube feeding.

The Breastfeeding Assessment Score is a tool to calculate whether a baby needs to have additional milk and how much. A 'full top up' is a full feed, and the amount of milk is often worked out by using the calculation 150ml x baby's weight in kg, divided by the number of feeds in 24 hours. For premature babies who may be struggling with weight gain this can be increased to 180ml/kg/day. A 'half top up' should be half this volume. Too often parents are told to top up with a full feed when the baby is actually feeding fairly effectively, which can cause babies to take too much milk. This means they may posset (when a baby spits up some milk after a feed) more, or they have to sleep it off and are difficult to rouse for the next feed. It is very important to keep top ups to a minimum wherever possible.

Score	Definition	Action
A	Offered breast, not interested, sleepy	Full top up (preferably expressed breast milk)
B	Interest in feeding, however does not latch	Full top up (preferably expressed breast milk)
C	Latches onto the breast, however comes on and off or falls asleep	Full top up (preferably expressed breast milk)

D	Latches, however sucking is uncoordinated or has frequent long pauses	Half top up – consider not topping up if mother is available for another breastfeed. Baby may wake earlier
E	Latches well, long slow rhythmic sucking and swallowing – short feed < 10 mins	Half top up – do not top up if mother is available for another breastfeed
F	Latches well, long slow rhythmic sucking and swallowing – long feed > 10 mins	No top up

Adapted from a scale used by Queen Charlotte's Hospital SCBU, London

For twins and triplets it is important to remember that they are individuals. One baby may be much better at feeding than another. It can be hard not to compare them, and be worried and frustrated if one baby is not managing to feed as well. But, with time, it is very likely that they will catch up and will feed well from the breast when they are individually ready.

Babies can be topped up with extra milk by cup, syringe, spoon, or paced bottle feeding. Many NNUs prefer to use bottles for top ups, and for during the night when the parent is not there. They are easier and there is less waste. However, there is a risk that the babies will develop a bottle preference due to the fast flow, as well as some premature babies finding the flow of the bottle overwhelming, meaning they may struggle to take a breath. Pacing the bottle feed allows the baby to have breaks and means they will be able to take control of the flow of the milk (Wilson-Clay 2005). An elevated side lying position can be very effective for babies struggling to bottle feed. Paced bottle feeding is discussed later.

Discharge home

Babies are often discharged somewhere between 36 and 42 weeks gestation. The breastfeeding parent and baby may be given the chance to 'room in' for a night or two before babies are discharged home.

During this time they are often encouraged to move on to more responsive feeding, as opposed to hospital routine based feeding. At this stage babies can still be sleepy and not wake for feeds so it is important to make sure that they are fed at intervals of no longer than three hours from the start of one feed to the start of the next. Once the babies are consistently waking before the three hours are up, then it is safe to move to responsive feeding. Some babies may still need additional expressed milk or formula when they are discharged home, which often means an intense 'triple feeding' routine of breastfeed, top up, and express every three hours or more, day and night. This is utterly exhausting and overwhelming and it can often be difficult to see past this stage. However, with good feeding support from health visitors, breastfeeding specialists and the neonatal outreach team, it is possible to move on to exclusive breastfeeding. Parents need to understand late preterm and early term behaviour, as well as full term baby behaviour and a feeding assessment should be carried out regularly to assess efficiency of breastfeeding.

PERSONAL STORIES
Joanne with Dylan and Oscar

At 25+3 weeks pregnant my waters broke while I was in the kitchen preparing tea. Deep down I knew it wasn't good. We raced to the hospital where they confirmed labour. Within hours, at 25+4 weeks, I gave birth to twin 1, a 1lb 10oz boy who we named Dylan. They had to work on him for half an hour to get him stable and I caught a glimpse of him in the incubator before he was rushed off to NICU. Our world had come crashing down and I couldn't believe what was happening. We all waited, fully expecting twin 2 to arrive, however, my labour stopped and twin 2 decided to stay put. The consultants said because twin 2 was in its own sac and had its own placenta they were happy not to intervene and to see what happened. They said I could potentially go full term with twin 2 although this was unlikely. I was closely monitored and bed bound in hospital, not allowed to see Dylan for fear of starting the labour process again so the nurses placed an iPad on top of his incubator so I could watch him from my room. Two days later on 12th January at 25+6 weeks labour started again and within a few hours twin 2 arrived, a second boy we later named Oscar. He weighed 2lbs. This time I heard him cry and then he too was also rushed off to NICU. I got to see them both for the first time later that evening and it was so sad seeing my tiny babies on ventilators fighting for their lives.

The boys were tube fed and on donor milk for the first few days until my milk came in. As they were born so prematurely I learnt about NEC [necrotising enterocolitis] – a devastating disease of the intestine mostly affecting premature babies. Premature babies who are formula fed are more likely to develop NEC than breastfed babies. To avoid this I knew how important it was for them to have my breast milk and as their Mum I felt it was the only useful thing I could do for them. So the pump became my best friend, with me expressing religiously every three to four hours, day and night, while at home and in hospital sat by their incubators.

For the first two weeks we prepared for the worst. They were so small and fragile and we had many ups and downs including brain bleeds and infections. We visited every day, did their cares, learnt how to test their aspirates and tube feed them. I was able to hold them together for the first time at nearly three weeks old and it was the best day of my life!

At 35 weeks gestation, with fab support from the NICU nurses, they learnt to breastfeed themselves. The bond doing this was incredible! Two weeks later we introduced bottles of my breast milk. The boys came home just before their due date and we had to adapt to home life with them being hooked up to oxygen and administering daily medications. I got into such a good expressing routine while they were in hospital that this continued to be our way of feeding alongside directly breastfeeding.

Victoria with Emelia and Elliot

I was admitted to hospital at 26+6 weeks where it was confirmed I was in early labour. With signs of fetal distress in twin 1, our world really was crashing down round about us. The on-call NICU consultant visited us and explained all the risks, the prognosis of twins born so early and asked me how I planned to feed them!

I had breastfed my eldest and always planned to try and feed the twins. That conversation was pivotal and I had no doubt that I'd feed my babies. Mums of preemies all sadly share the same feelings of guilt that we aren't able to keep our babies safe inside – but I knew that I could almost 'make it right' by pumping milk. And that's what I did! 8–10 times per day for 107 days. An emotional rollercoaster, and a lonely journey at times. NICU life is so busy, I was always there for all the cares, ward rounds, and investigations – expressing was integrated into this new routine. I was so fortunate to have an amazing milk supply which never faltered. We know how important mum's milk is for preemies and that was always my motivation, to help them grow and hopefully avoid NEC. Our twins had so many difficulties but took to breastfeeding so well, it was a slow gradual process that needed lots of patience (after three months in the NICU I was tired!) but we pushed on, and both babies came home after four months fully breastfeeding (with my little boy needing some high calorie milk to help him grow and help his lung development).

I always say that this is my biggest life achievement!

Lucy with Theo and Rory

At my routine 34 week scan my midwife took my sample and asked if I'd had any issues with my vision recently, or headaches. I replied not that I'd particularly noticed, but now that she'd mentioned it just that morning I'd seen some spangles but had put it down to being tired, given I was 34 weeks pregnant with twins and had been working until the week before! She informed me that there was protein in my urine and my blood pressure, having been very healthy at all other checks, was 'high for me'. I was whisked around to the day assessment unit, where they strapped me up to check the babies' hearts. I was then told my babies would be delivered the next day! I was in shock, I had not been expecting that news. They gave me the first of two steroid injections (ouch!) [to reduce the severity of lung disease of prematurity and of other associated complications for the babies] and told me to phone my husband to bring in my hospital bag – something else that wasn't 100% ready given I was not expecting to be having my babies this soon.

The next day I was gowned up and prepared for theatre for that evening. Both babies were head down, and I'd been hoping so much for a natural birth, but the consultants advised against it. They were concerned that with the stage of pre-eclampsia I had it wouldn't be healthy for me, or potentially for my babies, so a C-section was the way to go.

At 6pm we headed down and the spinal was administered. I remember very little after that point, I had a reaction to the anaesthetic so sadly didn't see them lift the babies out of me. All I remember is huge pressure on my ribs as they tried to move twin 2 down to get him out. My blood pressure had plummeted as had the babies', so they were urgently trying to get them out while bringing me back round.

The euphoria when I heard two little cries and my husband telling me we had two boys is like nothing I've experienced in my life. While the surgeon stitched me back up they took the babies to check them over and then brought them back to me wrapped up.

My biggest regret is not being able to put the babies to my breast immediately. But I spent that evening with the lovely nurses in the HDU [high dependency unit] hand expressing colostrum and feeding the babies with a syringe. The nurses from NICU were then concerned they weren't eating enough so took them away to NICU for the night to assess them, while colostrum was taken from me to give to them.

Unfortunately both boys lost a lot of weight, 13.2% and 11.8%, so they advised that the boys needed to be fed on a high calorie formula on a strict feeding plan to bring their weight back up. I was desperately trying to pump without much success in those first two weeks as I had always wanted to breastfeed. It was a long, painful, and worrying journey until I was able to fully breastfeed with the support of an IBCLC to help me. I did it, a whole year, and it will be something I'm eternally amazed about and proud of achieving.

Top Tips for Parents

Ask for a delivery room cuddle if possible. It may be a while before you are able to hold your babies again.

Hand express colostrum within two hours of birth, or as soon as possible. Ask for help with this.

Hand express every two to three hours, use a pump for extra stimulation if you wish.

As milk begins to 'come in' move to a hospital grade double pump.

Pump at least 8 times in 24 hours, pumping sessions do not need to be evenly spaced.

Pumping at night is incredibly important for milk production. Set alarms.

Massage gently before and during the pumping session. A hands free pumping bra is helpful.

Have something to remind you of your babies. Photos, videos, smell, sound.

Try a power pumping session once a day.

As soon as babies are stable and you are well enough, ask for kangaroo care.

Be as involved in your babies' cares as you can.

If babies show signs of rooting ask about trialling the breast. Ask for support with latching babies effectively.

Ask about risks and benefits of using donor milk, formula, fortifier, and any other decision around your baby's care so you can make an informed choice.

Ask questions, write a list as you think of them, if you do not understand something ask staff to explain and provide more information if they can.

Remember they are your babies.

When discharged home, make sure you have a hospital grade pump and accessories to use.

Make sure you eat and drink properly.

Do take some time off and do not feel guilty for doing this. Take some rest. Do one thing for you, it can be just having a coffee on your own for five minutes, or a bath, or a walk round the block.

Ask for support with everything at home.

Ask for support with assessing how the babies are feeding.

Discuss risk and benefits of different feeding interventions; tube feeding, shields, cups, bottles, supplemental nursing system.

As the babies become bigger and stronger and more able to breastfeed, try to be there for as many feeds as possible.

Take the opportunity to 'room in' before babies are discharged home if this is possible.

Remember sleepy premature babies turn into alert full term babies.

Early babies sometimes have a bit of a fussy period of frequent feeding somewhere around their 40 week due date, it can be a bit earlier or later. This often coincides with being discharged from hospital which can be quite unnerving!

— *Chapter 4* —

Late Preterm and Early Term Babies

A baby born between 34+0 weeks and 36+6 weeks gestation is defined as a 'late preterm' baby, while babies born between 37+0 weeks and 38+6 weeks are defined as 'early term'. The average length of a twin pregnancy is 36+4 weeks, with many twin babies born between 36 and 38 weeks gestation due to the NICE guidelines. This is considered full term for a twin pregnancy, but it is important to remember that the babies are not full term, and may have had another four to six weeks gestation had they been uncomplicated singleton pregnancies.

It is also important to point out that babies born earlier are also often discharged from hospital at around this gestation, and can experience similar difficulties with continuing to establish breast-feeding, after initially being fed expressed breast milk. All premature babies go through the late preterm and early term stage before they move on to feeding and behaving like a full term baby!

When surveyed in 2020, the parents in Breastfeeding Twins and Triplets UK Facebook Group cited birth between 36–38 weeks gestation as being the biggest barrier to establishing breastfeeding with their babies. Studies have also found that babies that are birthed at this gestation are less likely to go on to breastfeed, especially if they are born to first time parents (Hackman *et al.* 2016).

For babies who are born around this stage of their development, establishing breastfeeding can be quite difficult. They are often well enough to remain on the post-natal ward with their parents, but this can mean that they get treated the same as a full term baby and are expected to be breastfeeding responsively. Unlike parents of NICU infants who have used a breast pump to establish their milk supply by the time of NICU discharge, nursing parents rely more on the sucking stimulation of the infant to establish the milk supply.

The problem is that these babies often do not feed effectively or frequently, preferring to sleep. The fat pads in the babies' cheeks, which help to stabilise the breast in baby's mouth, have not yet developed. Research has shown that one third of infant brain development occurs in the last six to eight weeks of pregnancy. This suggests that neurodevelopmental maturation, rather than experience or learned behaviour, is largely responsible for feeding behaviours or late preterm and early term babies (Hallowell & Spatz 2012). Due to this immature brain development and suck pressure, they are more likely to be sleepy and hard to rouse, to fall asleep easily at the breast, to have short sucking bursts or to be uncoordinated in their 'suck, swallow, breathe' pattern, which is significantly associated with suboptimal breastfeeding (Meier *et al.* 2013). This can lead to real problems. Babies can have low blood sugar, lose weight, or develop jaundice. Milk supply may become insufficient, or it may be lost, even if established by expressing in NICU.

If the babies have been discharged without adequate follow up care in place, it is often decided at their next appointment that the babies need supplementing. But the lack of milk supply due to the babies' infrequent and inefficient feeding often means formula is needed. This then leads to a drop in maternal confidence and some will even wean entirely.

The first 48 hours

When babies are late preterm or early term, parents should be offered at least an hour of uninterrupted skin to skin after birth, as long as the birthing parent and babies are well, no matter whether the babies are born vaginally or by caesarean section. The staff will dry babies and place them on the parent's chest. The babies will be encouraged to latch and feed. This skin to skin time stabilises baby's heart rate, temperature, breathing, and blood sugar and encourages babies' natural feeding instincts (Bergman, Linley & Fawcus 2004). With twins, each breast will independently maintain the proper temperature for each baby (Ludington-Hoe *et al.* 2006). Babies are often quite alert in the first hour or so after birth and feed well, unless there have been lots of drugs in labour.

Routine hand expressing of colostrum alongside the babies breastfeeding, even if they appear to be breastfeeding well, can help protect against many of the early problems which may occur when initiating breastfeeding. If parents have collected some colostrum in pregnancy, this can be used to give the babies' blood sugars a little extra boost. The nursing parent can be supported to hand express a little after each feed so they have some extra colostrum to give. Not only will this mean the parents have extra colostrum to give to the babies, but it will also help to prime the prolactin receptors, and encourage the breasts to make a copious supply of milk.

It is essential to make sure these sleepy babies wake and cue to feed. Parents should be encouraged to feed no later than three hours from the start of the previous feed, thus ensuring a minimum of eight feeds a day (Nyqvist 2008). This will ensure babies maintain their blood glucose levels, and will keep the parent's prolactin levels stimulated.

Colostrum can be given if the parents are struggling to wake the babies to feed. As mentioned above, a little colostrum via syringe or finger feeding can boost the baby's blood sugars and give them the energy to then latch onto the breast and feed. Colostrum can also be given if the baby has had a short or inefficient feed to help them take a little more.

This should be standard practice for all babies at this gestation in our hospitals. It would likely reduce the need for early formula supplementation and increase longer term breastfeeding outcomes.

Breastfeeding in skin to skin contact encourages the baby's natural breastfeeding instincts, and encourages them to stay alert and feed more effectively. Getting into the routine of stripping babies to their nappies in these early days of breastfeeding can help them feed better. Many parents are unwilling due to having to disturb the babies to dress them again afterwards. It is true this can wake them up, but the parent can simply offer the breast again to settle the baby back to sleep, which will also help them take a little more milk.

Breast compressions can help, by massaging the colostrum down into the breast and making it easier for the baby to extract. We will cover this in more detail in the next section.

Ongoing breastfeeding

Milk begins to 'come in' around day 2–5, and many late preterm and early term babies find the increased flow will help them to be more efficient at the breast. Being mindful of the frequency and efficiency of the feed continues to be important, as some babies will still find feeding difficult, or may be a bit overwhelmed by the flow. If a baby is having issues with the initial strong let-down, alongside optimising positioning and attachment, hand expressing before the feed can stimulate the milk ejection reflex and once some milk has been removed, the babies may be able to feed more effectively.

Breast compressions

We all know that the baby sucking at the breast drives the flow of the milk. This happens in several ways, the vacuum caused by baby's jaw dropping, the massaging of the breast with the tongue, and the milk ejection reflex (or let-down reflex) triggered by the hormonal response to baby suckling.

However, the flow of milk also drives the baby's suck. A faster flow will keep the baby feeding actively for longer. Breast compressions can help increase the flow, and so encourage the baby to take more milk. This will lead to greater milk production, as more milk is being removed from the breast.

Breast compressions are the act of massaging and compressing the breast to increase the flow of milk. They may also increase the fat content of the milk, similar to the hands-on pumping technique mentioned earlier.

When doing breast compressions it is important not to disturb the latch by compressing too near the nipple, so the hand position is further back towards the chest wall than is usual when hand expressing. Fingers and thumb can be used to make a C shape around the breast, and a firm compression into the breast tissue and then holding for a couple of seconds is most effective. A good way to explain this to parents is to imagine the motion of squeezing icing out of an icing bag, as opposed to squeezing a spray bottle of cleaner, which is a much faster, lighter, and less effective. Parents who are tandem feeding can still do breast compressions, but a supportive feeding cushion or pillows will be necessary so that they can let go of the babies and use their hands. It is also possible for somebody else to do the compressions, but ideally it should be the breastfeeding parent as it is important to understand how firmly to squeeze to avoid causing pain or damage to the breast tissue.

There are two main ways to use breast compressions:

The most common scenario is when baby becomes sleepy and the gaps between sucking bursts increase. Doing a breast compression or two at this point will fill baby's mouth with milk, remind them they are supposed to be feeding and not sleeping, and prompt them to begin to suck more vigorously again. Often the baby will then maintain these stronger sucks for another few minutes. In this situation compressions can be used until they no longer cause the baby to restart active feeding.

Breast compressions are particularly effective for early term and late preterm babies with shorter sucking bursts. A short burst is something like 3–6 sucks before having a rest, compared to a full term baby who may do 10–15 sucks. It is immediately apparent that the baby with the shorter sucking bursts will be getting less milk over the same period of time, which can cause issues. Breast compressions can help extend these bursts of sucking – as the baby begins their sucking burst, the parent compresses the breast and holds for a few seconds. The baby will then do a longer burst of sucking before having a break, due to the faster flow of milk.

Supplemental feeds

If the babies continue to be sleepy or inefficient at the breast once the parent's milk has come in, the parent should be encouraged to pump between feeds in order to give some additional milk to the babies.

Top ups should always be kept to a minimum volume, and will not necessarily be required after every feed. A feeding assessment from an experienced breastfeeding specialist should be offered to assess milk transfer, and a realistic triple feeding plan drawn up involving the babies breastfeeding directly, being given extra milk (expressed or formula if supply of parent's milk is not sufficient), and pumping. Try to make the plan as efficient as possible using any help available. It is incredibly intense managing a triple feeding plan and should only be necessary for a short time. Getting the whole routine completed in as close to an hour as possible makes it more manageable, as this will have to happen every three hours.

Giving a baby additional milk can happen in several different ways using different equipment:

Syringe

A syringe works very well in the early days when small volumes of colostrum or milk are needed. A few drops at a time can be put into baby's mouth, or for a larger volume finger feeding can work well.

Finger feeding

A finger is inserted, nail down, into the roof of baby's mouth which will trigger their suck reflex. A syringe can then be inserted into the corner of baby's mouth and as baby sucks gently compress the plunger of the syringe. It is very important to go slowly and allow baby to swallow, as with too much volume baby is at risk of aspiration. A feeding tube placed along the finger attached to the syringe can also work well.

Spoon

A spoon suits small volumes of colostrum or milk. Sit baby upright with head back, chin off their chest, and place the spoon to baby's lips. Tip until the milk is level to the edge of the spoon, and baby should lap up the milk.

Cup feeding

Cup feeding is an effective way of feeding larger volumes of milk. Sit baby upright with head back, chin off their chest, and lightly swaddle so baby does not hit the cup and spill the milk. Place the cup into the corners of baby's mouth, tip the cup so the milk is level with the edge of the cup. Again, baby should lap up the milk.

Supplemental nursing system

If parents are still struggling and are finding they continue to need to supplement their baby, then a tube at the breast ('supplemental nursing system' or SNS), can be a great option. The tube not only delivers the top up the baby needs at the breast, so no need for bottles, but it also increases the flow of milk when baby is breastfeeding, thus helping the feed to be more efficient and stimulating the milk supply more effectively.

An SNS can be set up very easily with just a feeding tube and a bottle. The off-the-shelf ones can be a good option if the parents feel the system may work well for them, or if they need to supplement long term due to low supply. However, they can be expensive and a little tricky to use, so starting with a homemade version is often a good plan.

A French 5 or French 6 feeding tube is generally preferable. Take a bottle containing some expressed milk or formula. Some teats have an air vent in them which you can use to thread the tube through, or you may need to sacrifice the teat and make the hole bigger so it will take the tube. Feeding tubes often come with a cap and port so open the cap and place port into the milk. The other end of the tube should go into baby's mouth. Some find starting with the tube in place and then latching baby works best, while others find starting the feed without it and then inserting the tube once the baby is latched works better – either way takes a bit of practice. The tube needs to be far enough in to make sure baby seals around the tube and the breast, as if it goes in too far it may trigger the baby's gag reflex.

To change the flow rate of the milk the bottle height can be adjusted. If baby is struggling to suck strongly enough to draw up the milk then raise the bottle so that gravity will help. If baby is struggling with the fast flow, then lower the bottle. The shop bought ones are also adjustable.

You can also use feeding tubes with a syringe by fitting the syringe into the port. Very gently compress the syringe as baby is feeding – often just resting your thumb on the plunger is enough pressure. If tandem feeding, one tube can be used for each baby. It is probably best to have two separate bottles to keep an eye on the babies' individual milk intake.

To use the SNS, start the feed just on the breast and use some compressions to keep baby feeding actively. Once baby slows down or becomes fussy at the breast, either insert the tube or take baby off and re-latch with the tube in place. Continue the feed with the supplement flowing through the tube. The increased flow of milk will encourage baby to feed more actively again, and they are likely to trigger another milk ejection from the breast too, which will help increase supply.

To clean: hot soapy water, syringe. Flush hot soapy water down the tube, followed by clean water to rinse. Feeding tubes should not be heat sterilised as this degrades the silicone. Cold water sterilising can be used, but may degrade the silicone more quickly. Tubes need to be changed regularly and should be inspected frequently for cracking or discolouration.

A tube at the breast is not for everybody. It is a bit of a faff and can be a bit tricky to clean. However, it is important for the option to be discussed and it can be incredibly useful if long term supplementation is necessary.

Paced bottle feeding

All babies having bottles, whether they are exclusively bottle fed or also breastfed, should be given their bottle using the paced bottle feeding technique. Pacing the bottle feeds slows down the flow of the milk and gives babies breaks, which serves several purposes. With traditional bottle feeding the milk flows so fast that the baby's 'suck, swallow, breathe' pattern may not be possible, and they end up sputtering and choking. The fast flow also doesn't give the baby time to realise it is full. The hormone Leptin is linked to feelings of satiety, telling our brains when we have eaten enough, but if baby is still receiving a fast flow of milk they don't get a chance to notice this sensation of fullness. This can then mean they are either sick and bring it back up again, or they are so full that they are difficult to rouse for the next feed. Not to mention that if the parent is trying to express for this bottle then a baby taking so much can be very disheartening.

Pacing the feed means that the baby will take less wind, as well as reducing the risk of overfeeding by giving the baby a chance to realise they have had enough. When combination feeding, paced feeding also lessens the likelihood of flow preference and breast refusal, so it's very important that anyone giving a bottle is shown how to give it in this way.

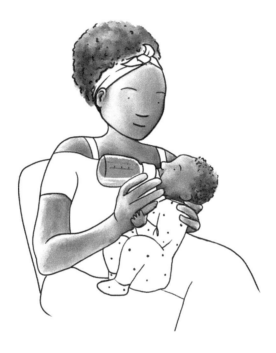

In order to pace a bottle feed, baby should be sitting fairly upright but with head tilted back off the chest. Start by brushing the top lip with the bottle to invite the baby to open wide, just as they would to latch onto the breast. Insert the teat into the roof of the mouth and allow baby to suck with no milk present. They will not swallow the air, and doing this will encourage the baby to wait for the let-down reflex when feeding from the breast. After 30 seconds or so, tip the bottle up so the tip of the teat is full but the bottle is as horizontal as it can be – this will keep the flow slower. Once the baby has drunk some milk, tilt the bottle own again and let them suck on an empty teat for a few sucks. This gives them a break, and an opportunity to let you know if they've had enough milk. After this break, tilt the bottle back up and fill the tip of the teat again. If baby needs a total break then take the bottle out completely and wind baby. It's important to make sure you do not try to make the baby take more than they need, even if there is milk left in the bottle. They will show you when they have had enough – perhaps by turning their head away, or pushing the teat out of their mouth with their tongue, or by holding their hands up.

Triple feeding routines for twins

Triple feeding is incredibly intense, overwhelming, and often quite confusing when there is more than one baby, so having a gentle routine can help to ensure each baby has a turn on the breast while also receiving the milk they need. Here are some scenarios that can work well:

Single feeding with a helper

Breastfeed first baby, watch for active feeding, use breast compressions to encourage baby to take more milk. Pass to helper to top up. Breastfeed second baby, watch for active feeding, use breast compressions. Pass to helper to top up, then pump for the next feed.

Single feeding without a helper

It can be a good plan to try to encourage babies to be out of sync so the whole triple feeding routine can be done with one baby before starting the other. Of course this does not always work! It is possible (though tricky) to top up one baby while breastfeeding the other. Try to pump when finished.

Tandem feeding with a helper

Breastfeed both babies, watch for active feeding and use breast compressions to encourage babies to take more milk. Either the helper gives the top ups to both babies in tandem while parent pumps, or each take one baby to top up and then pump afterwards. To tandem bottle feed the helper will need some way of propping babies up a little (feeding cushion, bouncy chair, lap etc.) and use a bottle in each hand. It is more difficult to pace the feed when tandem bottle feeding but sometimes needs must!

Tandem feeding without a helper

Breastfeed both babies, watch for active feeding and use breast compressions to encourage babies to take more milk. Top up both babies using tandem bottle feeding. Pump afterwards.

With a hands-free pumping bra and some practice, it is sometimes possible to pump while giving the bottle top ups.

How to tell if baby is feeding effectively

Some babies will be ready to fully breastfeed at 36 weeks gestation, others at 42 weeks, or at some point in between, or, for some babies, even later. Understandably where there have been weight gain concerns it is common for parents to continue to supplement and schedule far longer than necessary due to being cautious. However, triple feeding is incredibly time consuming and overwhelming, so we need to move away from it as quickly as possible in order for parents to find breastfeeding a sustainable option.

If each baby is putting on weight as expected, doing plenty of wet and dirty nappies, generally waking themselves for feeds before the three-hour schedule, and having a good proportion of 'active feeding' during a breastfeed, then top ups can be gradually phased out, and it is safe to move on to responsive, cue-based feeding.

Ideally each family would be guided by somebody highly qualified, such as an IBCLC or Breastfeeding Counsellor. This is a scenario that deserves specialist breastfeeding support in the home on discharge from hospital, to ensure the babies' breast milk intake is maximised. Unfortunately, in reality parents are often left to get on with it by themselves, with no clear plan in place.

Once the babies are more efficient at feeding from the breast, there are a number of stages we can go through to move towards exclusive breastfeeding. Babies should also be weighed regularly throughout the process to make sure they are still roughly following their curve on the growth chart.

First we need to make sure baby is going to the breast every feed. If a feed is missed because of giving a bottle, milk production will decrease. When milk is left in the breast it sends messages to the milk producing cells not to make any more, but if the breast is emptied frequently the production goes up. The more you feed, the more you make. If baby will not go to the breast for a feed, or if parents would like to keep one bottle feed for a break, then milk should be expressed instead. If baby is fussy at the breast and not feeding well for a feed, expressing should be encouraged to boost supply.

It is important to put baby to the breast during the night. It might be tempting to skip a feed and get some sleep, but this can be detrimental to milk supply. Prolactin, the milk making hormone, is at its highest at night so we want to take advantage of this to put in an order of milk for the next day and help maintain a full milk supply. Again, if baby is not coming to the breast, or the nursing parent is finding breastfeeding at night unsustainable to begin with, it is essential that milk is removed by pumping instead.

If baby is having a high volume top up after every feed (more than 30–40ml) but is now feeding efficiently and putting on weight steadily, the first step is to drop the volume of formula in each top up. Your baby will probably start doing this naturally themselves as breastfeeding becomes more efficient, so follow their lead. However, because of the fast flowing nature of bottles, and the baby's suck reflex, they will often take more milk than they actually need from a bottle, as discussed previously. It is essential to pace any bottle feeds.

When a smaller volume is given in the bottle, baby may be unsettled but can be put back on to the breast to settle if necessary. This will trigger another let-down of milk, which will help boost milk supply, and also encourage baby to get used to settling in this way. Parents could also be encouraged to express after the feed if the baby has settled, or if the baby will not go back onto the breast, in order to increase supply. However, pumping is often the thing that is most unsustainable, so prioritising baby feeding directly is often more effective at increasing supply.

Babies should be encouraged to feed frequently, watching for the earliest feeding cues such as stirring, hands to mouth, rooting, head nodding. Parents can try to enable a feed as soon as they see these.

If baby is still a little sleepy and not waking for feeds then it is still a good plan not to let baby go longer than three hours from the start of each feed.

It is a good idea to clear the diary, get a feeding station set up with everything the breastfeeding parent needs: snacks, drinks, phone, remote control and some good box sets to watch, and do as much feeding and skin to skin as possible. I like to call this 'Topless Telly Time'. It is often referred to as a 'Baby Moon'.

Once the baby is on a small volume top up every feed, it may be time to drop some of the top ups completely. It is important to get baby weighed to ensure weight gain is steady and has not slowed due to the decreased top ups. If weight gain has slowed, it may be a case of waiting a bit longer to start decreasing or to reintroduce some more milk and maybe pump.

Babies will often settle after the breast more easily at certain times of day. Mornings are often a good time to try without a top up. Babies tend to feed well, settle easily, and there is often more milk available at this time. Baby can be encouraged to feed frequently or cluster feed during this time until they have had enough. After a day or two, milk supply will have caught up and baby should be more settled. Then the period of no top ups can be extended, or a top up can be dropped at another time of day. Night time is often another good time to stop top ups, as after the first few weeks of life, babies will often have a nice calm feed and go back to sleep fairly easily. Late afternoons and evenings are often the most unsettled time for a baby and so parents often stop these top ups last, although it should be noted that this natural tendency to want to cluster feed can be very useful to boost supply.

Tandem feeding can be very helpful during these periods of frequent feeding as it can mean parents can respond immediately with a feed for both babies rather than one having to wait for the other to finish.

Another option for working on dropping top ups is to pump after every feed and work to replace formula top ups with expressed milk. This technique will be necessary to increase milk supply if the baby is not efficient at the breast and is consequently not transferring the milk well, or is too sleepy to take a whole feed. As the babies become stronger and more able to feed, they will be able to take more milk directly and pumping and topping up can be gradually reduced.

Parents may get to a stage where they are at maximum capacity for breastfeeding, whether there are physiological reasons, or perhaps just that they find exclusive breastfeeding is too much. In this scenario combination feeding can be a good option. It's very important that parents are aware that it doesn't have to be all or nothing – all breast milk the babies receive is beneficial to their health and that of the nursing parent.

PERSONAL STORIES
Helen with Robyn and Marley

My MCDA girls were born at 36+2 via C-section. The epidural failed, so we had to convert to an emergency section, which led to some trauma and not getting the birth I had hoped for. My wife was only allowed in for two hours a day due to restricted visiting times for infection control, so for 22 hours a day it was me trying my best. Both babies really struggled to latch and my milk came in on day 7. The babies were losing weight, and the hospital spoke to me about the potential for needing nasogastric (NG) tubes, which, isolated in hospital, felt terrifying. Triple feeding commenced, but with some staff saying start three hours from start of feed and others saying from the end of the feed [Note: it is recommended to not let newborn babies go longer than three hours from the start of one feed to the start of the next]. I had advice to only allow a latch for 10 minutes, and other advice that it is imperative to allow baby to spend time at the breast each time for as long as they want.

It was a whirlwind of back and forth, pressing the button, pumping, top ups, until we were discharged a week later. I left 20ml of expressed milk in my hospital bay and sobbed my heart out until my wife ran from the carpark back to scoop it up! The most crucial thing I realised was that they are my babies, and it's my body and my choice. We stopped filling the babies with top ups like we were making foie gras, and when it felt right to ditch the book of colour coded statistics, ease the pressure off, and eventually to just responsively breastfeed, it was the most liberating feeling. Blebs, blisters, blocked ducts, vasospasm, and mammary constriction syndrome punctuated my experience in the early days, which I wouldn't have gotten through without the support of an amazing breastfeeding peer supporter and post-natal doula, as well as the fantastic support of Breastfeeding Twins and Triplets UK Facebook Group. One year down the line I feel insane pride and gratitude for what we have achieved!

Elizabeth with Clementine and Charles

We had a straightforward delivery and both babies latched on soon afterwards. They seemed to be feeding well so I was told that we could go home from hospital the day after they arrived. I was overjoyed! But a couple of days later when the community midwife visited she said the babies looked jaundiced and they'd lost too much of their birth weight, so we had to be readmitted to hospital. It came as such a shock and absolutely floored me. Having been happily back at home with the support of my family, suddenly I was alone in the hospital with both babies on bright blue sun beds undergoing phototherapy for jaundice.

Thankfully the infant feeding lead was just finishing her shift and came to see us after she was meant to have gone home. She immediately diagnosed tongue tie in my boy twin, which she dealt with there and then, and put us onto a strict three-hourly schedule of triple feeding. But by the time I'd breastfed both babies, syringe fed them my expressed milk and then pumped again for the next feed it was almost time to start the cycle again, so sleep and rest didn't really feature in those few days. It was brutal, totally unsustainable, and felt like it would never end. I hit an all-time low with the combination of hormones, sleep deprivation, and both physical and emotional exhaustion, but I kept going.

After two days like this we were allowed home again. The babies were still struggling with weight gain though, so I bought a pump and implemented my own triple feeding scheme where my husband gave the babies their top up syringe feeds while I pumped, enabling me to squeeze in that essential bit of rest between feeding cycles. Eventually we got to a point where I was able to phase out the top ups and just nurse them direct.

I wish that someone had warned me about all of this either when I was opting to have a C-section at 37 weeks or as we were being discharged from hospital the first time. Those early days would still have been intense, exhausting, and challenging, but foreknowledge is empowering.

Top Tips for Parents

Try to do some antenatal hand expressing if you get the go-ahead from your health care professionals.

Have immediate skin to skin with your babies if possible, either both together or birth partner can have one and you have the other.

Encourage a breastfeed within the first hour after birth.

If babies do not latch, or are too sleepy to feed, hand express some colostrum. They can be given this by syringe. You could also use any colostrum which you have hand expressed ante-natally, but if doing this it is important to also hand express to give your breasts the stimulation.

Encourage babies to feed, strip them down to their nappies, have skin to skin; if they are sleepy give them a little hand expressed colostrum to boost blood sugar levels.

Wake babies to feed if they are sleepy. They should be feeding a minimum of 8 times in 24 hours which is roughly three hours from the start of each feed to the start of the next.

Ensure babies are latching deeply. Ask for support with this.

Use breast compressions to help babies take more from the breast.

Hand express between feeds so you have some extra to give if they need it, and so your breasts are stimulated frequently to help future milk production.

As milk begins to 'come in' use breast compressions to help babies take more milk.

Wake babies after their first go on the breast at each feed, and encourage them to have another go.

Keep an eye on nappy output. A baby should be doing at least two poos a day from birth.

Ask for support with feeding once you are discharged. Your infant feeding team or local breastfeeding support may be able to help. Or you could book an IBCLC (Independent Board Certified Lactation Consultant).

If babies are not feeding effectively, try to express your milk after each feed so you can give it as a top up.

If babies need top ups, see if someone can help you with the supplementary feeds while you breastfeed and pump.

Top ups should be kept to a minimum wherever possible. A full feeding assessment and plan should be offered when discussing topping up.

Top ups can be given by syringe or teaspoon if a small volume, cup or paced bottle if larger volumes.

Remember this triple feeding routine should only be temporary! It is very intense and difficult to maintain.

If formula is necessary this does not mean that you will not be able to exclusively breastfeed long term. Think of it as a medicine to help your babies to breastfeed – this is what it was originally designed for.

Ask for support to move away from top ups once babies are feeding more effectively. It should be possible to move towards exclusive breastfeeding if that is what you wish.

As soon as babies are generally beating you to the three-hour wake up, you can relax and follow their lead. Remember most babies prefer to feed more frequently.

Early babies sometimes have a bit of a fussy period of frequent feeding somewhere around their 40 week due date (although it can be a bit earlier or later).

Sleepy early babies turn into alert full term babies! Try to view this as a positive even though it can be quite intense.

— *Chapter 5* —

Full Term Multiples

Full term is defined as a baby born between 39 weeks and 40+6 weeks. Twins born full term or close to full term, and some early term babies who are alert and coordinated, can feed just like a full term singleton from the beginning. But we have to remember that all premature and late preterm and early term babies will also develop into full term babies. Most babies go through a similar pattern of development, although the exact timing of this development varies from one baby to the next, even from one twin to the next. Babies born a bit early are even less predictable. But all babies smile, sit, move, and walk in the end (assuming they do not have underlying health problems).

The first feed
Just as for babies born at late preterm, when babies are born at full term or early term, parents should be offered at least an hour of uninterrupted skin to skin after birth (see 'The first 48 hours' in Chapter 4).

For a vaginal birth there is often a longer gap between first and second baby arriving and this can be a lovely time to have skin to skin with twin 1. There may even be time for a feed. Once the contractions start up again the birthing parent may want to pass the baby to their birthing partner to continue skin to skin while the second baby is delivered.

For caesarean births the birthing parent's gown will be worn loosely and heart monitors placed out of the way to leave room for a baby. Skin to skin can be done in theatre while the parent is being stitched back together. It is a nice distraction! Or, if preferred, skin to skin can be started back in the recovery room once the procedure is finished.

The birthing parent can have skin to skin with both babies and try a tandem feed as their first feed if they wish. They can ask the staff for support with this. Or they can have them one at a time to do skin to skin and feed and the birth partner can have the other. Whichever twin seems the most keen to feed should be given to the birthing parent, but it is worth warning the birth partner that their baby will likely try to latch on! As soon as one twin has fed they can swap. This skin to skin time with the babies is really lovely and can be a time for the parents and babies to start to get to know each other, as well as being very calming for everybody.

Once babies have had a rest after birth, they start to show some feeding cues, licking lips, head bobbing, putting their hand to their mouth, and beginning to search for the breast. If they are left to their own devices they will often find their way to the breast themselves and latch on. The parent can encourage a little by lifting the breast a bit or helping them shuffle along. This can also be done with both babies in tandem with a little jiggling. Babies are hardwired to find their first meal. If they are allowed to put these instincts to use and then feed well for the first time, they are likely to be able to do it again later in the day, after a bit of a snooze! There are lots of videos of 'the breast crawl' online which are lovely to watch.

If the birthing parent or either baby is not well then they can have skin to skin whenever they are able. This does not mean they will not be able to breastfeed. If one or both babies are taken to the neonatal unit they can have skin to skin, often known as kangaroo care, as soon as they are stable and the parents are able to visit. This golden first hour can be recreated as soon as possible and will still trigger the baby's feeding instincts.

If the breastfeeding parent is unwell, their partner can have some skin to skin time. It is very important to remember that skin to skin and kangaroo care is not just for the birthing parent. Fathers, partners, siblings, and grandparents can all partake and it is beneficial for all.

If the babies do not latch on and feed in this first hour or two (for whatever reason) then it is really important to hand express colostrum so that the babies can have some from a syringe or feeding tube. This will give the babies food, energy, and antibodies, and will help to kickstart milk production. If the babies continue not to latch then hand expressing should be continued every two to three hours and the colostrum given to the babies. Parents can ask for support to help babies to latch – sometimes it can take a bit of time for it to work. Protecting milk production while baby learns to latch will ensure that breastfeeding can still be established later, and babies can benefit from the mother's milk.

We would expect a baby to do at least one good size dark green/brown/black sticky meconium poo in the first 24 hours after birth and one wet nappy. Urate crystals are the norm at this stage and parents should not be alarmed to see them.

The second night

Once the babies have had their first feed they may be quite sleepy. It is hard work being born! This can be a good time for the birthing parent to rest, but it can also be a time when the parent is actually full of adrenaline and cannot sleep.

Full term babies should start to wake more regularly for feeds after a few hours. It is important to follow the babies' lead and feed responsively. However, some new babies can be quite sleepy and, if they haven't woken themselves for a feed after three hours has passed from the start of the last one, it is a good idea to wake them with a nappy change and encourage them to feed. If baby is struggling to wake or they are too sleepy to latch effectively, the parent can hand express some colostrum, or use previously harvested colostrum, and syringe or finger feed it to the babies. This often boosts the baby's blood glucose levels and they have more energy to feed effectively. If the babies are waking more frequently then feed at the earliest feeding cues, when baby is just stirring, licking lips, sucking hand, and wriggling a little. Crying is a late cue and babies may need to be settled first before they can latch effectively.

Colostrum is available in small quantities and it is perfect for baby's small tummy, but they need to refill regularly! Most full term babies like to feed somewhere between 8 and 12 times in 24 hours, so it is important for parents to understand that frequent feeding is to be expected and is, in fact, a very good thing.

On day 2 we would expect to see two wet nappies and two good sized poos. They will probably be quite dark in colour but may be beginning to lighten a little. This is a good sign baby is getting enough milk.

On the second night babies often really start to wake up, and usually have a bit of a feeding frenzy. We call this behaviour cluster feeding. We think it is partly to do with encouraging the parent's milk to 'come in' in abundance, but also that baby has realised they are no longer cuddled up safe in the uterus and are out in the big scary world. The parent's chest is a safe place: the source of safety, warmth, and food. This is home! So this is where they wish to be, feeling and smelling their parent and hearing the same heartbeat that has been their constant companion for the past months. This can be quite difficult if the birthing parent is still in hospital and the birth partner has had to go home. Support from the hospital staff will be key.

Babies often spend several hours repeatedly going back onto the breast, taking some more colostrum each time. It may also be related to the recent findings in a study that the volume of colostrum when hand expressing reduces after the first 12 hours, and then increases again after 30 hours (Kato *et al.* 2022). Of course the volume a baby can take directly is no relation to what the parent can hand express – babies are generally more effective – but it may encourage the baby to want to feed more often. And, of course, the more frequently a baby latches and feeds in the first few days, the greater potential for future milk production due to priming the prolactin sites. Supplementation should not be necessary if the babies are feeding effectively and being fed responsively. This cluster feeding behaviour often catches parents by surprise, but it is very common and doesn't mean anything is wrong, although it can be very challenging with more than one baby. Tandem feeding can be beneficial.

Babies generally lose a little weight after birth. Up to 7% is considered normal weight loss. If babies have lost 10%, a clinical assessment of baby should take place and feeding observed by a person with appropriate training and expertise. If a baby loses more than 10% or has not returned to birth weight by three weeks of age, then a referral to paediatric services should be considered. If baby is not feeding effectively, prioritise the use of expressed milk. If supplementation with infant formula is necessary, encourage expressing and feed the infant with any available human milk before giving any formula (NICE 2017).

Early babies once they reach 40 weeks gestation

For those babies that are born early, we often find that around 40 weeks gestation babies begin to wake up and behave more like full term babies. This can happen a bit before or after 40 weeks – all babies are different – but they will all do it at some point. Anecdotally we have noticed in Breastfeeding Twins and Triplets UK Facebook Group that there seems to be a bit of fussy behaviour around 40 weeks for these babies where they suddenly start to want to feed more frequently, cluster feeding behaviour begins and the babies do not settle as easily. So they display similar behaviour to the second night for full term babies. This makes total sense as I believe this behaviour is developmental. This can be quite unnerving for parents who have just been discharged home with their babies, especially for those parents who have had babies in NICU and are used to hospital routines and scheduled feeds. This is where education around normal newborn baby behaviour is essential.

This can be a great time to really focus on breastfeeding if the babies have been struggling a little, as they become more alert, waking more frequently for feeds and are highly motivated to want to go to the breast! If supplemental feeds are being given this can be a good time to begin moving away from the triple feeding routine. Frequent and efficient breastfeeding usually boosts milk production more effectively than pumping.

PERSONAL STORY
Holly with Finn and Solly

I'd had three previous singleton full term births (two at home) and found it very frustrating [when expecting the twins] that consultants kept telling me I should be induced at 37 weeks. I held them off until 39+1 when I was going in for a routine scan. It was a bank holiday weekend, my mum was staying at our home looking after the others, and I knew that my previous births had been very quick so was worried about doing the journey from home in labour, and I found myself saying yes to the offer of having my waters broken. They were broken at 11am and my husband and I went to eat lunch in the hospital canteen. We walked around and I got annoyed at nothing happening and started regretting saying yes. Then at about 2pm I felt period-like cramps so we went back up to the labour ward.

At 2.30pm, although I kept saying I was fine, my swaying and demeanour must have looked familiar so my husband called in the midwife. As soon as I saw her my contractions went mad and I knew the first baby was coming. She got me on the bed on all fours and Finn arrived at 2.55pm weighing 7lbs 1oz. I held him for a minute and then knew number 2 was arriving. A consultant burst into the room and demanded I lie on my back to scan his position despite me saying I needed to be on all fours quickly, but it was too late and I could feel baby moving down. The wonderful midwife held my leg up and told me to go for it. She filled me with confidence and I began pushing against her.

Thankfully by this point the head consultant was in, she saw his bum arriving first and ordered everyone to stand back and not touch him. After what seemed like an age his head came out, he was blue but she was reassuring as she put him on my tummy and allowed the cord to keep pumping for a few moments to help oxygenate him. Sonny was born at 3.07pm weighing 6lbs 9oz. He was taken away quickly to be given oxygen but was back within a few minutes. That night a midwife showed me how to tandem feed lying back and even took a photo for me saying I should be so proud of myself. I felt like superwoman!

I know we were incredibly lucky to have a brilliant hospital and midwives who encouraged breastfeeding so that combined with my determination to do it meant there was no question of ever doing anything else.

Top Tips for Parents

Immediate skin to skin after birth.

Babies' natural instincts should enable them to latch themselves onto the breast if placed on the parent's chest.

If immediate skin to skin is not possible because babies are unwell, have it as soon as possible.

If immediate skin to skin is not possible because the birthing parent is unwell, the birth partner can have skin to skin.

Please do not worry if immediate skin to skin does not happen, you can do this at any time. It does not mean you will not be able to breastfeed. It just helps to get things started.

If colostrum has been harvested, this can be given by syringe if the babies cannot feed directly, for whatever reason.

Encourage babies to feed frequently. If they do not wake themselves by three hours after the start of the last feed, wake them. Eight feeds in 24 hours is the minimum a baby should be fed.

If babies are struggling to wake, some expressed colostrum can be given to give them more energy to feed, hand expressing after each feed if necessary.

Breast compressions can help them take more colostrum.

Babies only need small quantities of colostrum in the first 48 hours.

Cluster feeding behaviour on the second night is very common and normal. This will help your milk 'come in' in abundance.

Babies should be doing at least two poos in 24 hours from birth. Stools will become lighter in colour from black tar-like meconium to brown, then green and by day 6 they should be mustard yellow. Seedy bits are common.

Babies should be doing one to two wet nappies on days 1–2,

three or more on days 3–4, and five or more on days 5–6. From then on at least six wet nappies a day. Urates are common in the first couple of days. If you aren't sure how to tell a nappy is heavy/wet then add 2–4 tablespoons of water to a nappy and this will give you a good idea.

Ask for support from the hospital staff, especially if feeding is painful. They will help you and the babies to get a deep latch.

Milk usually begins to 'come in' on day 2–5.

Triplets

0.02% of pregnancies in the UK result in triplets, so it is incredibly rare (Multiple Births Foundation 2019). The average gestation for triplets is 34 weeks, and the majority will be born by elective caesarean section, and almost all will spend some time in the neonatal unit.

The journey to exclusive breastfeeding or combination feeding is largely the same for triplets as it is for premature twins, with a few additional considerations. So please start by reading previous chapters on premature birth and early term birth for an overview of feeding. The main considerations for triplets are that milk production needs to be higher as there is an extra baby, and the logistics of feeding three babies with only two breasts. There is little research into the possibility of making a full milk production for three babies, but there are certainly several examples of parents managing to exclusively breastfeed triplets in the Breastfeeding Twins and Triplets UK Facebook group. Parents will often need extra support in the early days as caring for three babies is a mammoth task no matter how they are fed!

Here are some feeding patterns that breastfeeding triplet families use:

Exclusive breastfeeding/parental milk feeding

Tandem feed two babies and single feed the third afterwards; rotate which baby has the single feed.

Tandem feed two babies and bottle feed the third with expressed breast milk – with practice the breastfeeding parent can feed all three at once this way. Pump after the feed for the next one. Rotate which baby has the bottle of expressed milk.

Single feed all three babies. Some parents prefer this, and as the babies become more efficient on the breast this becomes a more realistic option.

Some will do a combination of direct breastfeeding and expressing, perhaps having the other parent or a helper do one or two feeds a day with only pumped bottles so the nursing parent can get a stretch of sleep.

Combination feeding with formula or donor milk

Tandem feed two babies, bottle feed the third, rotate which baby has the bottle feed. The breastfeeding parent can feed all three babies at once with this method.

Single breastfeed one baby each feed, and bottle feed the others.

Breastfeed most feeds and bottle feed all three babies for one or two feeds a day to give the breastfeeding parent a break.

PERSONAL STORIES
Alexa with Elvie, Iris, and Fletcher

It's hard to know where to start in describing our breastfeeding journey. I can't praise the nurses in SCBU enough. They had nothing but admiration and encouragement for breastfeeding my triplets, and luckily, because the babies didn't have any health challenges, I was able to do this from very early on. Having said that it wasn't all plain sailing: after a large blood loss and a stressful and unexpected transfer of hospitals my milk didn't 'come in' until day 7 really. In the meantime I had to allow the babies to be given formula. I hadn't heard of donor milk at that stage and no one suggested it. I really hadn't wanted them to have formula so young, but the doctors said they needed the calories and I felt I had no choice. However, from the pumping I managed to give them at least some of my milk, and very quickly they weren't having formula at all. They all latched early on but one baby was better than the others. The nurses also suggested we get them used to bottles too and occasionally, especially with my littlest baby, we still had to tube feed and add fortifier. So they fed three different ways for three weeks, but they were always fine at whichever method we used.

We were in SCBU for those three weeks, and by the end of this time all babies were exclusively breastfed with a little fortifier for one. It was exhausting to be honest, and if I'd been sent home earlier I am not sure I'd have been able to sustain the pumping as well as feeding, but the support in SCBU helped me to do that. Once at home I hired a hospital grade pump and still expressed once or twice a day for a little while but this was more because I was paranoid about not having enough supply. The hospital had put the babies on a four-hourly feeding schedule, slightly staggered. This started to blur a little bit when we got home but largely worked out, and enabled me to feed them separately during the night. I think I was really lucky in that all my babies only fed for about 15 minutes at a time so it was manageable to feed all three, and mostly to feed them separately. I never really got into a habit of tandem feeding but did use it as and when I needed to. I'm so proud to have been able to give them this start in life and proud to be able to say I exclusively breastfed triplets (after the first week). It's one of the greatest achievements of my life really.

Chapter 6

Tandem Feeding

With twins, there are two babies and there are two breasts. Many twin parents like to feed their babies together to save time, which is commonly known as tandem feeding. Tandem feeding can be started as early as the first feed, or parents may find they prefer to try it later on once the babies are feeding more effectively and the parents are more practised. It is useful for all multiple birth parents to be able to tandem feed, so offering this as part of breastfeeding support is great. Some parents choose not to tandem feed for all sorts of reasons, and it is important to point out it is totally possible to breastfeed multiples without tandem feeding, especially as they get bigger and more efficient.

Pros of tandem feeding

Tandem feeding synchronises the babies' feeding times and more importantly can help synchronise their sleeping times as well! Babies can be encouraged to feed together. When one baby begins to stir the parents can wake the other and offer a feed to both. Once this is quite well established, babies often begin to wake naturally at the same time.

Being able to tandem feed empowers the breastfeeding parent to feel that they can cope with two babies on their own. One of the most stressful parts of having to look after two babies alone is needing to settle both at once. Being able to tandem feed makes this much more doable. This is especially useful if the partner has to return to work.

There is often one baby who is a stronger feeder than the other.

Tandem feeding means that the strong feeding twin can help a weaker feeder by stimulating the let-down and getting the milk flowing. Their more vigorous sucking can drive the flow of milk meaning it is easier for the weaker feeder to take more milk.

Tandem feeding also increases milk supply and weight gain. Research shows that milk yield is greater, and is higher in fat, when double pumping (Prime *et al.* 2012), so we could assume the same for tandem feeding. When a parent single feeds the milk ejection reflex happens in both breasts, and often the milk in the breast that is not being fed from leaks. Tandem feeding means all the milk is used. If single feeding, the milk goes unused until later meaning it is left in the breast slowing production. Tandem feeding also makes it easier to feed the babies responsively. When parents can only single feed, one baby often has to wait which can result in babies coming to the breast less frequently overall.

With a good breastfeeding cushion or support parents can breastfeed both babies with their hands free, so they can feed themselves, use the remote control, or help older siblings.

PERSONAL STORY
Kath with Drew and Jevan

I was shown how to tandem feed by a very helpful midwife, the day after my babies arrived. She went and found some extra hospital pillows and we made a nest around me and managed to position the babies so they could latch well. That was it! I knew that if I could feed the babies together I would be ok. When I was discharged home it took a bit of practising with our home cushions on our sofa. I got a bit sore as I was struggling to keep the babies latched deeply and it was making my wrists ache, but I kept at it and things improved. I tended to wake the second baby as the first was stirring, although they actually got in sync quite quickly. Sometimes one would need a second or third go on the breast and in this scenario I would single feed.

When the babies were about three weeks old my partner and I took a walk to our local breastfeeding support group. I could not believe my luck – one of the supporters was also a mum of twins, breastfeeding her 18-month toddlers. She lent me a twin feeding pillow to try. I have to say it was a total game changer and supported the babies at a good height, even if I let go to eat my dinner! Tandem feeding really helped me cope and also get some sleep. I did get a little obsessed and would get stressed if one baby fed at a different time from the other, but it always worked out ok and I could convince them to feed together again.

Cons of tandem feeding

It can be more difficult to latch the babies with only one hand – although a tandem feeding cushion can help with this. In the early days when babies can take several goes to latch trying to deal with two popping off the breast can be quite stressful. First time parents who are less confident with handling babies may find it more challenging.

For some tandem feeding positions it is necessary to use both hands, or both arms, to support the babies, which means it is difficult to do anything else. It can feel very overwhelming and parents can feel trapped and unable to move; it may feel quite claustrophobic. They cannot get up and move when they are tandem feeding. Sometimes parents report feelings of wanting to escape.

Tandem feeding can increase feelings of nursing aversion. Nursing aversion is a phenomenon that some breastfeeding parents experience, which includes having particular negative feelings, often coupled with intrusive thoughts, when an infant is latched and suckling at the breast, making them want to stop the feed. It has been noticed that it is more common with tandem feeding, whether that be two babies of the same age, or an older child and a younger baby. These parents generally do not want to stop breastfeeding but may need strategies to help them cope with the aversion (Yate 2017).

PERSONAL STORY
Sarah with Lowri and Caelan
I did some tandem feeding during the cluster feeding times in the early weeks. After that I single fed for pretty much the rest of the

first year. I returned to some tandem feeding after that at their request. They would shout 'Do 2, do 2!' at me!

Single feeding meant I could walk around, answer the door, let the dog into the garden, get a drink or snack, do something for my older child, and not feel trapped. It does take more time. But it is a viable option.

How to start and positions

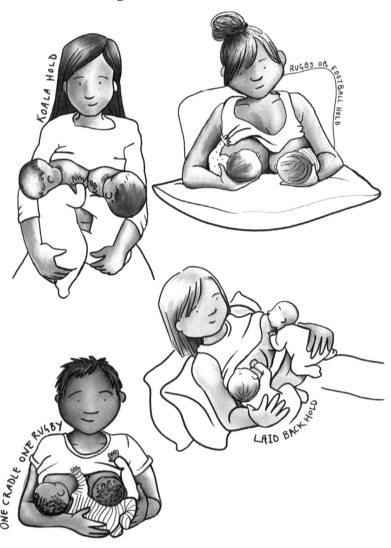

Some parents will be given the opportunity to do a tandem feed as their first feed. If babies are both alert and rooting after birth they can be encouraged to have skin to skin together, and go on the breast. Otherwise parents may prefer to latch each baby separately to start with.

Later on it really depends on how the babies are feeding and how confident the parents feel about latching babies on together. Some babies struggle to latch in the early days so trying to juggle two babies and latching both on with one hand each can be quite stressful. And they often take a few goes each to latch. So sometimes it's preferable to wait until they have practised feeding singly, especially for parents who are not yet confident handling babies.

Some babies, especially if they are full term, are a good size, and are nice and alert, can tandem feed straight away. Some try tandem feeding and just don't enjoy it, and that's fine too. Only the breastfeeding parent can decide what works best for them. However, it's always a good idea to be able to tandem feed if they need to, even if they don't do it all the time. The babies will at some point both wake up hungry simultaneously, and it can make dealing with cluster feeding much easier.

Double rugby/football hold

The most popular position for tandem feeding is the 'double rugby/ football hold'. The parent will need to get everything set up in advance, not forgetting to grab a drink, snack, and their phone, and make sure the remote is within reach! A sofa or bed is generally more successful, as chairs are often too narrow to take both babies and feeding pillows.

Begin by lifting both babies into position. If the parent has to reach for the second baby, the first will probably come unlatched. If there is a helper, they can pass the second baby once the first is latched. The babies lie down each side of the parent, starting nose to nipple with chin on the breast, so the babies need to be quite far back with their legs curled round the parent's waist; they may need an extra cushion or two in behind their back to make room for the babies' legs so the babies don't kick off the sofa.

Support the baby with a hand behind their shoulders, with thumb and fingers round the neck behind the ears. Tickle the top lip with the nipple to stimulate baby's rooting reflex so they open their mouth wide, and bring on to the breast chin first with nipple going up into the roof of the mouth. Then try to do the same with the second baby. The parent should try not to twist or move too much when latching the second baby or the first one will just come off and they will have to start again. This can happen frequently in the early days.

Some prefer to latch the more difficult feeder first so that they can concentrate more and use both hands. Others prefer to latch the easy baby first, get the milk flowing and then latch the second baby. Then if the first comes off, they can re-latch the easier feeder. There are no rules, parents can do whatever works for them.

Twin feeding pillows

A twin feeding pillow can help to support the babies in a good position. If the feeding pillow is set up well the adult should be able to let go of the babies and feed hands free.

Twin cushions come in two shapes – U-shaped and W-shaped. With all U-shaped twin breastfeeding cushions make sure the parents are sitting upright and push the cushion right in so there is no gap by their tummy. Most brands come with a back support cushion, which should be used, possibly with the addition of another cushion to make sure there is enough room for the babies' legs to wrap around behind the adult's back. The cushion should bring the babies to exactly the right height to latch on to the breast. If the babies are not high enough the cushion can be lifted by adding a pillow underneath, or the parent can sit on a softer surface so their bottom is a bit lower relative to their knees. If the cushion is too high they could try sitting on a cushion, or on a harder surface like a firm sofa. A cushion that is too high is quite difficult to use, so it's generally better to choose a lower option and adjust upwards.

For the W-shaped cushions, place them in W position behind the parent's back. Fold the two outer sides down on either side of the parent, and if there is a clip fasten it in front. Some of the cheaper cushions do not have a clip, and in this case it may be a good idea to sew a ribbon or fastening to the ends to prevent the cushion from splaying out sideways. If the pillow is too low to support the babies in a good position then the parent could try placing a bed pillow on their lap and resting the sides on top of this. Sometimes it may be necessary to add some cushions under the sides too.

Some may prefer to use bed pillows, a pregnancy cushion, beanbags, and/or sofa cushions. There are many options and it does not matter what is used as long as the babies are supported in a good position to feed, and that the parents are not hunched over the babies to feed. It is very important that the parent has sufficient lower back support and brings the baby to them rather than leaning down to the babies as this can cause neck, back, and shoulder issues.

Parents often need a different set up in bed than they do on the sofa due to a different sitting position and often a softer surface. It can be a good idea to try to work on the bed set up for a daytime feed – trying something new at 3am is never a good plan!

Many breastfeeding parents are worried about how they will be able to tandem feed without help when their partner goes back to work. The most important thing is to keep everything nearby within reach. Get the feeding pillow (or other cushions etc.) organised ready. Pick up one baby and put on the sofa or bed next to where they will be feeding. Ensure baby cannot roll or push themselves off. It is surprising how early babies can move themselves! Then pick up the second and place next to the first. Get settled and make sure the feeding pillow is in position. Then they lift one baby onto the pillow, ensure they cannot roll off, either using an arm to support baby, or some prefer to roll up a muslin or blanket and place behind the baby's back to stop them rolling. Lift second baby onto the cushion. Babies can be lifted one-handed using 'kitten hold'. This involves taking a good handful of the front of the babygrow or sleep suit and lifting gently. The neck of the clothing supports the baby's neck and the baby can be lifted carefully over short distances. This poses little risk as long as done slowly.

For babies who are often sick, or suffer from bad wind or reflux, it is possible to tilt the cushion a little so babies' heads are higher than their hips. Putting feet on a footstool to lift knees a little and then lean back a bit can make more of an angle, or sitting cross legged or with knees bent on the bed. This means the angle of the cushion and the adult's body is still the same but the babies' heads are elevated, which makes them less likely to get trapped wind.

Other tandem feeding positions

Parents do not have to be constrained by the double rugby/football hold and the need to use a feeding pillow. There are several other positions they could try. As the babies get older, have more head control, and faster at feeding, they really can be quite creative. Here are a few:

THE STACK

Commonly called 'The Stack', this position involves feeding one baby in cradle hold and one in rugby hold. This is quite a good position for feeding out and about as it can be done either without a cushion at all, or with just a couple of cushions to support the parent's arms. A changing bag or a rolled up coat can also be used to support the baby in rugby/football hold, or the parent can sit cross-legged on the floor and use their legs to support the babies.

DOUBLE CRADLE

The 'double cradle' can be another good way of tandem feeding without a pillow. It is especially useful when babies are a bit older and can feed in a more sitting up position. The babies' legs go between the parent's legs and they are cradled in the parent's arms, one on each side, with the parent slightly reclining so their body takes the babies' weight.

DOUBLE KOALA HOLD

In koala hold the babies sit astride the parent's legs facing inwards. If they are not quite at the right height the parent can raise or lower their knees for small adjustments. This position can be good for babies who have reflux or lots of wind, or for babies who struggle to maintain a deep latch. It is more difficult if parents are short, or if breasts hang quite low, so doesn't work for everyone.

DOUBLE LAID BACK POSITION

The laid back position involves the parent reclining on some pillows at about 45 degrees, and the babies lying on their tummies on the parent's body. Usually in this position babies can self-attach. This is often a position that parents use for their first feed and is the position babies will instinctively bring themselves to after birth. It's a good position for babies who have reflux or lots of wind, or who are struggling to get or maintain a deep latch, perhaps because of a tongue tie. If the babies are refusing the breast for any reason this position can reawaken the natural breastfeeding instincts of the baby, especially when starting in skin to skin. As with koala hold, it is more difficult if breasts hang quite low.

TANDEM FEEDING IN THE SLING

If a parent can master the 'tandem twin sling feed' then they can feed walking around – the ultimate food on the move! A long, structured wrap, two ring slings or one of the twin specific slings can be used. Finding an experienced sling consultant can be very empowering as there are so many options.

TANDEM FEEDING LYING DOWN

Possibly most importantly, there are ways to tandem feed lying down so the parent can lie back and relax while they feed. These positions can be used from birth when babies like to feed very frequently, or later on during the long cluster feeding sessions when babies are going through periods of brain development or growth spurts. Double laid back position can work well. Side lying position for one baby, with the other lying along the parent's side or draped across parent's back or front is another option. A laid back version of The Stack sometimes works well. These are all options that can be tried. Parents can get quite creative – nipples are circular after all, so babies can latch from any direction.

Of course, when the babies become toddlers they can feed any old how. Upside-down, standing up, all sorts of gym-nurse-tics!

Top Tips for Parents

Don't be afraid to try tandem feeding.

Ask for support in hospital.

Take your feeding pillow to hospital but leave it in the car. They are bulky so carrying them around to different departments will be difficult.

You can do a double laid back position as your first feed if you wish. Or you can feed them singly if you prefer, or if there is a big gap between babies arriving.

Some prefer to tandem feed straight away, others prefer to leave it until they are more confident and babies are feeding well. There is no right way to do this. It is whatever works better for you. You can do a bit of both if that suits you.

Make sure babies are latching well and transferring milk effectively. If worried, your infant feeding team or local breastfeeding support should be able to help, or you can book an IBCLC (International Board Certified Lactation Consultant) to visit your home.

Tandem feeding can help in the evenings when cluster feeding is common.

Being able to tandem feed, even if you do not choose to do so all the time, is empowering as it means you will be able to cope on your own if both babies are unsettled.

If using a twin feeding pillow, make sure it is the correct height for your body shape so that it supports the babies without needing to stoop. The cushion should not be too low or too high.

There are many different tandem feeding positions to try. Get creative!

— *Chapter 7* —

Breastfeeding Continued...

New baby behaviour

Although each baby is an individual, full term babies have patterns of behaviour and development that happen at similar times. It can be useful for the parents to understand normal baby behaviour, so that they know whether something is wrong. Having a group of families, whether face to face or online, with similar age babies can be reassuring for parents when many of the babies are doing the same things as theirs. However, it is important to remember that if the babies are born a little early they will often reach developmental milestones a little later. And, also, all babies are different!

For babies born prematurely, these developmental stages often seem to happen somewhere between actual age and adjusted age. So the babies will still go through each stage, but possibly not exactly when the guidance predicts they will. They often begin to catch up as they go through the first year, and officially health care professionals stop correcting for prematurity at age two.

Daytimes

Once the sleepy first few days or week or so are over, babies often start to display some common patterns of behaviour. Young babies are often a bit more settled in the mornings, so this is a great time for parents to stay in bed and catch up with some sleep, try to catch a shower, or to pump if they are still doing some bottles, as it is often easier to get a larger volume of milk at this time of day.

As the day wears on, babies often start to feed a bit more

frequently, often every couple of hours or more and, by the time the evening arrives, the cluster feeding kicks in!

Evenings

Babies are often much more alert in the evenings and first part of the night than any other time of day. They can also be quite unsettled. Cluster feeding behaviour is common, where babies want to feed very frequently, going back onto the breast over and over again. Parents often worry that their milk has run out as their breasts can feel soft and the milk flow slows, but milk continues to be available for the babies. Each time they go back onto the breast the milk ejection reflex is triggered and more milk is released. Milk is being made in the background all the time, even while the babies are removing it, so there is always some available.

Sometimes babies start to reject the breast after a few goes, but are still unsettled. Again, parents often believe it is because they have run out of milk. But in my experience it often means that babies actually want to suck for comfort but do not actually want any more milk. So they latch on, suck, the milk arrives so they come off. Offering a clean finger to suck can help, or if parents are choosing to use a pacifier, this can be a good time to offer it.

There are also many other things to try during these fussy periods. Skin to skin, rocking, patting, swaying, tiger in the tree position, using a sling, massage, bath, sucking a finger, going for a walk, or even a trip in the car! After a bit of time trying some other things, offering the breast again often works and hopefully baby will settle.

Some parents will offer a bottle and the baby seems to take a large volume of milk and then crashes to sleep, which of course continues to fuel the self-doubt around milk supply. The problem is babies love to suck. A bottle teat is a firm stimulus, and when put into the roof of a baby's mouth, their suck reflex will be triggered. They have no choice but to suck it. And the flow of a bottle is very different to that of a breast, even a gentle suck will make the milk flow quickly. When baby's mouth is full of milk their swallowing reflex will make them swallow it, the teat hits the roof of their mouth again and the cycle repeats. Once they have taken all this extra milk that they did not really need, they are so full that they just fall asleep to recover. Think Uncle Bob after Christmas dinner! Offering a bottle is not a good test as to whether baby is still hungry. They will almost always take the milk, even when already full.

Nights

After these cluster feeding 'witching hours', babies often have a longer stretch of sleep. This can be a good time for the parents to do the same! This is likely to be the longest stretch of sleep, so taking advantage of this helps cope with the rest of the night. As the night progresses waking for feeds may become more frequent. Many babies like to cluster feed in the early hours of the morning, and are often more difficult to put back into their sleep space at this point in the night, so safe bed-sharing can be a good option, or parents may take turns to cuddle babies and stay awake.

The safest place for babies to sleep is in a cot by their parent's bed, however bed-sharing in a prepared bed is a much safer option than risking accidentally falling asleep with babies in an unsafe place, for example on a sofa.

It is important to remember that night feeds are essential for making a full milk supply. Prolactin, the milk making hormone, is at its highest in the early hours of the morning and removing the milk during this time helps with supply the next day (Wambach & Spencer 2021). If the parents are having to give bottles in the night, for whatever reason, it is imperative that milk should be removed by pumping instead or it can be difficult to establish and maintain supply.

Coping with broken sleep

Parenting and feeding more than one baby during the night can be very demanding. But there are a few things which parents can do to make it easier to cope.

Parents could consider co-bedding the babies in the same sleep space. There is some evidence that twins or triplets who share a sleep space may show more synchronous sleep states, and so wake at a similar time, which can make night waking easier to deal with (Ball 2007). I believe twins often settle a little better if together, although there is little researched evidence of this.

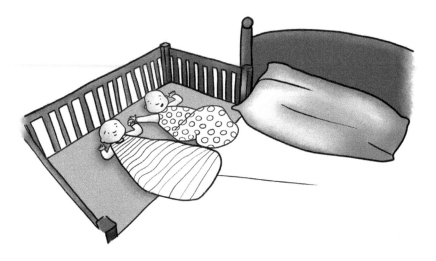

Keep the babies close to the parents. A large co-sleeper cot, or a cot with the side taken off attached securely beside the bed, can be a great option. Babies can be reached and settled back to sleep without the parent even getting up. As it is often the act of lowering a baby into a cot that wakes them, being able to feed and then roll away or slide them sideways can make a big difference. Co-bedding twins or triplets can encourage parents to keep the babies in their room for longer (which is recommended for SIDS prevention up to six months) due to reasons of space and ease (Ball 2006).

Some parents find it helpful to introduce other sleep associations alongside feeding to sleep, which can help the babies to be a little more flexible if feeding does not work. These can include shushing, stroking, patting, rocking, white noise.

Tandem feeding two babies takes the same amount of as time as feeding one, so many parents will wake the second baby if the first starts to stir and feed both. Once this routine is established, babies often begin to wake themselves at similar times, especially if co-bedded. This can maximise the gap between feeds and so maximise sleep. However, some people find settling the babies after tandem feeding more difficult and so prefer to single feed. Others prefer to single feed so that they can feed lying down more easily. As discussed earlier, there are some tandem feeding lying down positions that the parents can experiment with – though some may be easier when the babies are a little older. Each individual baby in a set of multiples may have quite different sleep needs to their sibling(s), so it can be beneficial to let them wake themselves. There is no correct answer to this.

A simple bedtime routine can help the babies to understand it is night time. The circadian rhythm (the baby's body clock) is governed by the secretion of melatonin in response to dim light (Akacem, Wright Jr & LeBourgeois 2016). Melatonin, a hormone released at night that is associated with the sleep–wake cycle, begins to be secreted from around one month of age, but does not reach stability until around three months (Biran *et al.* 2019). In the early days a bedtime routine can be as simple as lights dimmed, change of clothes and a feed to sleep. Some parents may like to add a bath or massage into this too, but it is not necessary. Sometimes it can be less stressful to bath babies at a different time of day when they are less tired. Breastfeeding helps the circadian rhythm develop as there is more tryptophan, the chemical precursor to melatonin, in human milk in the evening and night than in the daytime (Acuña-Castroviejo *et al.* 2014). Plenty of exposure to daylight in the daytime helps to cement the circadian rhythms. Ideally naps should be in light conditions with normal levels of noise unless the baby is particularly sensitive.

Safe bed-sharing can help when the babies are unsettled. Both babies should be on the side of the bed with the breastfeeding parent. A bedside cot with mattress level to, and pushed firmly against, the bed can help make a bed 'extension' if more room is needed. Some families will move the partner out of the bed so that the breastfeeding parent and babies have more room. Sharing a bed with a baby is the biological norm and what humans do around the globe. But it is important to remember to do it as safely as possible. The Safe Sleep Seven is a good guide:

1. Nobody in the household should smoke. Smoking increases the risks of SIDS.

2. Parents should not bed-share if they have drunk any alcohol

or taken any drugs or medications that may make them less aware.

3. Breastfeeding is protective against SIDS.

4. Baby should be healthy and full term. There is no research on when it is safe to bed-share with a premature baby. The parents will have to make their own informed decision on this. They should certainly avoid bed-sharing in early infancy.

5. The baby should be lying on its back when not breastfeeding.

6. The baby should be in its own bedding and dressed in layers to reduce the risk of overheating.

7. The bed should have a firm, flat mattress with bedding and pillows kept out of the way of the babies. Pack any cracks (e.g. between the bed and a wall) to make sure babies cannot get stuck, and make sure they will not fall off the bed. Again, this is where a bedside cot with a mattress at the same height as the bed can work well (Wiessinger *et al.* 2014).

Babies sometimes will not settle when put down, even right next to the parent, preferring to sleep on the chest of an adult. There is no research to say that this is a safe way to sleep, so it may be best to stay awake in this scenario. Tag teaming with the other parent, or an adult helper, may make this more doable in order to get a stretch of sleep without babies on them.

Many parents decide to introduce one bottle into their daily routine in order for the breastfeeding parent to achieve a longer stretch of sleep. Once milk supply is established this can work well, as missing a feed at the end of the day often has less impact on supply. Offering a bottle feed of expressed milk as the last feed of the day means that the other parent can give this bottle without it impacting too badly on their night of sleep, so work is possible the next day. The breastfeeding parent can go to bed early and get a stretch of sleep, having expressed this milk at some point earlier in the day. Some express as the last thing they do before sleeping, others will express the following morning when it is often easiest to get a good amount. It is often necessary to pump more than once in order to get enough milk for both babies, as it may not be possible to get enough in one session. Pumping at a similar time every day will help the breasts make more milk, as the body is getting the message that the babies need an extra feed at around that time. Parents may decide that they would prefer to give a bottle of formula so they do not need to pump, and in this case it is important that they have conversations about the risks of introducing formula to milk production and to gut health in order to make a fully informed choice. There is no evidence that formula will make the babies sleep longer than expressed milk or direct breastfeeding, although this is a myth parents often hear.

Again, it is very important to remember that if the parent thinks that they may fall asleep when feeding their babies that it is far safer to do so in a safely set up bed than it is on a sofa or armchair. Sofas and armchairs are never a safe place to sleep with a baby.

Partners can help massively even if babies are fully breastfed. Although many people get fixated on helping by feeding the babies, actually getting up with the babies in the morning before work and letting the breastfeeding parent sleep can give them another, very valuable, hour or two of rest. Staying up with the babies in the late evening while the breastfeeding parent goes up to bed can also make a big difference, as can getting up in the night to take care of nappy changes etc. and bringing the babies to the breastfeeding parent to be fed. Taking babies out for a walk in the daytime to enable a nap can also be useful.

Sleep is not a linear progression. Every time a baby goes through a growth spurt or leap in development, sleep can be affected. Lyndsey Hookway states in her book *Let's Talk About Your New Family's Sleep*:

> ...you will notice periods of increased sleep disturbance around times of development. It is almost as if the baby is investing so much energy and thinking power into learning something new that any new habits you are trying to establish with sleep go on hold. The human body is wonderful at prioritising tasks... I often say to parents that trying to make changes to sleep during a developmental phase is like trying to redecorate while you are having building work done. It is often easier to make changes once the dust has settled. (Hookway 2020, p.94)

Most babies continue to need milk in the night for the first year and beyond. Seventy per cent of babies aged 6–18 months wake 1–3 times a night, and mostly need a night feed (Hysing *et al.* 2014). There will be periods of more settled sleep, but there will also be times where they seem to be up every hour.

Breastfeeding is by far the quickest and easiest way to settle a baby (and the parent) back to sleep, and it is the biological norm, so there is no need to stop this. There may be phases where this method does not work as well, and then other ways of settling may need to be used, but this is normally temporary. It can be useful to overlay some other sleep cues so that sometimes somebody else may be able to settle the babies – this can include slings, cuddles, rocking, stroking, white noise, singing, music, smells of the parent, and all sorts of things.

Babies do not need to learn to self-settle or self-soothe. Being able to go to sleep independently is a developmental stage which they will all do eventually. Just like walking and talking, the age where a child is able to regulate themselves and settle back to sleep without adult support varies widely. Some will be able to do it at quite a young age, others well into toddlerhood and beyond. Some children may be able to settle if they have no immediate needs, for example hunger, thirst, warmth, being uncomfortable, or not feeling secure. Night waking is normal through toddlerhood and beyond. Adults often wake two or three times in the night, it is just that we are able to respond to our own needs, regulate ourselves, and settle ourselves back to sleep.

PERSONAL STORY
Ruth with Samuel and Naomi
Sleep became very tricky around four and a half months. This is a completely normal developmental phase and shows that they are learning lots of new skills, but it was extremely difficult with twins! I generally prefer to tandem feed, but with such frequent waking I preferred to feed them lying down in bed to maximise my dozing time. A few things really helped us get through the increased night waking. First we have a bed which is set up for safe co-sleeping. Next to our double bed is a cot bed with one side

off that is attached with cord to the bed frame, and the mattress pushed right against our bed with noodle floats (under the sheet) down the gap against the other side of the cot bed. This means the babies have their own space, but I can simply slide them to and away from me to feed in the night as needed. I have the double bed which allows me to tandem feed safely sat up with the tandem pillow if necessary. Second I have taken any opportunity to nap in the daytime when I can. This means weekends when Tom is around and some weekdays when my parents have come over, even just an hour in the day makes me feel better. The babies nap well in the slings for Daddy and grandparents too while I nap. Third I find with breastfeeding that I get back off to sleep much more quickly after being woken than I have done in the past when not breastfeeding. This is down to the hormones involved. So, if I'm going to be woken up, I like the fact I drop off again as soon as they settle. I think that aspect would be much harder for me if I wasn't breastfeeding because I know I find it hard to fall asleep again if woken abruptly.

First few weeks

Ideally, babies should always be fed responsively, watching for the early feeding cues (stirring, licking lips, hand to mouth) and aiming to feed them before they cry. Crying is a late cue, and a crying baby is likely to need to be calmed down before they are fed. If the babies are sleepy, it can be a good plan not to let them go longer than three hours from the start of one feed to the start of the next, in order to ensure a minimum of 8 feeds in 24 hours. However, most newborn babies like to feed more frequently than this. As soon as the babies begin to consistently wake before the three hours are up, parents can relax and feed responsively.

Cluster feeding is normal behaviour. Most babies like to cluster feed, and it is often at night to begin with. Babies do not begin to develop their circadian rhythm (body clock) until they are several weeks old, and having usually been more active in the womb at night, they tend to continue this pattern when they are out!

It's important that for all feeds the breastfeeding parent ensures the baby's latch is deep, and watches for active sucking and swallowing. A feed can vary in length from 5 minutes to 45 minutes – just like adults, babies sometimes want a large meal and other times just a snack. There should be deep jaw movement, sucks, and swallows, consisting of bursts of sucking with gaps in between.

Babies should be encouraged to have a second try on the breast at every feed. A nappy change after the first go can wake baby up, and then they are quite likely to want to feed again. If tandem feeding, parents can put each baby back onto the same breast. The more vigorous suckling now baby is alert will trigger another let-down of milk and baby will be able to take some more. This can be a good way to help ensure the babies get a good amount of milk in the early days. Later on babies are often fine with just one go on the breast.

Nappy output: ideally we would like to see at least six wet nappies a day from day 6 and at least one meconium poo a day in the first couple of days and two good sized poos a day from day 3 (UNICEF 2022). After around six weeks some babies may not pass a stool every day, but as long as there are plenty of wet nappies and everything else is going well, this can be normal. Before six weeks a feeding assessment would be a good plan to ensure baby is getting a good amount of milk, as a lack of stooling may be a red flag for poor milk transfer.

Feeds should be comfortable, although parents may experience some initial latching-on pain. If the pain only lasts for the first 15–20 seconds and the rest of the feed is comfortable this can be normal. This pain will stop happening after the first few weeks. If the breast-feeding parent is experiencing pain, pinching, or rubbing throughout the feed, then encouraging them to seek breastfeeding support is a good plan.

Fourth trimester

We call the first three months or so the fourth trimester. There are three trimesters of pregnancy, and the fourth is a period after birth where babies continue their development outside the womb.

As discussed in Chapter 2, humans are 'carry' mammals, as are all the apes and also marsupials. A bit like a kangaroo's joey, a human baby, if placed on the parent's stomach after birth and left to its own devices, will crawl up to the parent's chest and then latch themselves on to the breast. This is called the 'breast crawl' (as described in Chapter 5). The baby then expects to be fed very frequently. Other primate babies are more developed at birth and cling to their parent's fur. Unfortunately humans do not have fur or a pouch, but we can make an approximation of a pouch by using a sling or carrier. A baby's natural habitat after birth is the chest of the lactating parent. Here they will find warmth, safety, security, and a source of nutrition. For millennia around the world, human have been creating pouches with fabric in the form of a sling or carrier, so that they can easily carry their babies, nurture them, keep them safe, and meet their needs.

Growth spurts and fussy behaviour

Babies go through periods of more frequent feeding and fussy behaviour, during which they frequently really don't like to be put down! Often called growth spurts, we may be able to see an increase in baby's physical growth after a period of frequent feeding, but it is often fuelled by a leap in development as well. It is not that the parent is not making enough milk for their babies, though this is a common worry. It is better to see it as the babies feeding more frequently to ensure that they make enough milk. The more the babies feed, the more milk is made.

There are fairly consistent times when babies show this behaviour, including at around three weeks, six weeks, three months, and then regularly every couple of months after this. However, it is important to remember that all babies are different – in fact a set of twins may experience these fussy periods at different times from each other, and they may deal with these fast periods of growth and learning in different ways. In addition, premature or early babies may take a little longer to reach their developmental milestones, and the timing can be quite variable.

It can be tempting to reach for the bottle during these times, but they are temporary and should only last a day or two, or a few days, and then the babies will settle down again. If a bottle of formula or previously stored expressed milk is given the breasts will not get the message to make more milk and it will take longer for milk production to catch up with what the babies need.

Days when babies are fussy and feeding frequently can be challenging. To ride it out nursing parents can surround themselves with everything they need, plenty of snacks and drinks, get the TV on, and feed, feed, feed: Topless Telly Time! This is a great moment to call in those favours – ask for help with everyday tasks, or if someone could watch the babies for an hour so the parent can have a nap or take a shower.

At around three weeks evening fussiness can start to develop. It is commonly known as the Witching Hour; in reality it can be a couple of hours at least. The night time cluster feeding usually subsides and babies begin to settle a little easier at night, but it moves earlier to the evening, just as parents are exhausted from the day and trying to eat their dinner!

We are not sure why this happens. Milk flow may be a bit slower. It may be about baby destressing from a busy day, or perhaps they are overstimulated and are finding it difficult to regulate. They often love to cluster feed. However, the babies may get to the point where they no longer want to latch but are still not settled. Many tired parents think that they have run out of milk at this point but milk production happens in the background all the time so breasts are never empty. It maybe that baby is actually full of milk but is still awake, is tired and unsettled, and it is almost impossible for them to self-regulate.

Things parents can try when cluster feeding stops working are, in no particular order: rocking, patting, sucking finger, baby-wearing, massage, bath, tiger in the tree position, bounce, going for a walk, or going for a drive. Once the baby has had a little break they will probably latch and feed well again, and hopefully settle to sleep.

This time of day is when parents often opt to give a bottle, especially with multiples, as it is so challenging to deal with when there is more than one baby. The babies have often been cluster feeding for hours, they get given a bottle and they take a large amount. This further fuels the feeling of low supply at this time of day. The firm stimulus created by the bottle teat into the roof of baby's mouth forces them to suck – this is a reflex action. Babies find it difficult to control the flow of the milk and cannot just suck for comfort from a bottle, so they often take a large volume even if they do not really need it.

Giving a bottle at this time can help a fussy baby settle and, if the parent can pump for this evening bottle, their milk supply will be protected. Pumping once or twice or more at another time of day will produce the extra milk that the babies take in the evening. This can be a good option if this fussy period is proving difficult to manage, but it can be hard to find the time in the day to pump and sometimes the babies still prefer to be settled on the breast after the bottle, so this is a personal choice for the family to consider.

Coping and mental health

It is really important to remember that humans are not designed to parent alone. We are designed to parent in extended family groups, villages, tribes. Traditionally this is what human society looks like. This social structure involves lots of help and support for the new mother – somebody to cook and clean and provide food, and to take the babies when the mother needs to sleep, or to feed the babies. Traditionally lactating sisters, cousins, aunts, and grandparents who had breastfed in the past would re-lactate, and would help to feed the babies, especially if there were any milk supply issues.

From an evolutionary point of view, our babies still expect to be born into this world. But modern society has seen more families being split, spread across the country or even the world. Families have to parent in isolation without the support of extended family. Parents have to return to work. Our society is just not set up well to make it easy. Is it any wonder that post-natal depression is on the increase?

There are support options out there for families, but they can be hard to find or cost money. Many families who have relatives nearby will have some support, but grandparents and adult siblings are often working, so their availability can be limited. If a family has any sort of budget then some paid help can be incredibly useful. A post-natal doula can help look after the breastfeeding parent and support with looking after the babies. Maternity nurses are common in more affluent multiple birth families, they tend to take over looking after the babies, so it is essential to find somebody that has good breastfeeding knowledge and understanding of normal new-born behaviour. A 'mother's help' can help around the house with cooking, cleaning, and a bit of childcare. A clean house is one of the more difficult things to maintain while looking after several small humans, so a cleaner can make a big difference. There are volunteer organisations that can offer support for a few hours a week, which can sometimes be very useful if getting out to groups is difficult, or for spending time with older children.

Baby groups can be a daunting prospect with more than one baby, but a group that is set up well and accommodating to multiple birth families can be a real lifeline. As a parent of multiples, it can feel as though you are a bit of a freak show, and sometimes parents with singletons find it difficult to relate to the difficulties of having more than one baby but, normally, once they are used to it, they have nothing but admiration. However, twins clubs are places where the other parents truly understand the challenges, and these friendships can last for years. I still meet up from time to time with other twin parents from my local twins club to this day.

Online communities are also incredibly valuable. Being able to have a moan at 3am when the babies have woken for the billionth time, and to have someone reply with solidarity from another part of the country is very comforting. It helps parents to know that they are not alone in experiencing this! It is essential that online spaces are moderated effectively to ensure there is no spread of misinformation, but when they are evidence-based in nature, they are invaluable.

The thought 'If only I had one baby' will pop into the minds of most multiple birth families at some point during their parenting journey, often then making them feel incredibly guilty for these feelings. We need to acknowledge that these feelings are genuine, reasonable, and actually unsurprising. Nobody plans a multiple birth. Adjusting to the reality of having more than one baby at once can take time. These feelings can sneak up on parents when they least expect it – when one baby is wanting to be fed and the other is crying for a feed, when one needs a nappy change but they are dealing with the other, when one is being helped to sleep more than the other, when one just needs more attention, it is common to grieve for that one to one relationship they would have had with one baby.

Multiple birth parents are continually spread very thin and torn in multiple directions, especially if older siblings are also involved. They can constantly feel that they are not enough.

However, it is also important to remember that multiples get a lot of comfort from each other. They always have someone to snuggle up with. They have a constant playmate. And also someone to fight with! It is a very special and unique relationship which is fascinating to watch. An adult twin once said to me that she never noticed the fact she got less attention from her mum than her singleton friends, but she did realise that she had a very special relationship with her twin sister.

If parents are struggling with mental health, it is very important to seek help. They can make a doctor's appointment and be referred for counselling, or medications can be trialled. There are several safe anti-depressants which can be taken while continuing to breastfeed. Some people may suggest stopping breastfeeding, but numerous studies have shown us that breastfeeding protects maternal mental health, and that not doing so when it was your goal to feed your babies in this way can be very detrimental to mental health (Kendall-Tackett, Cong & Hale 2011). Breastfeeding cessation is a risk factor for increased anxiety and depression. Although some women will take comfort in the message that what matters most is that baby is fed, or 'fed is best', others view such suggestions as a lack of recognition of their wishes and of the loss that they feel, exacerbating their grief and frustration (Brown 2018). Stopping can also cause low mood due to the changes in balance of hormones, especially oxytocin. Justine Fieth wrote in an article for La Leche League UK:

> There is little research on the topic, but we know that the hormones so important in breastfeeding – prolactin (milk making hormone) and oxytocin (the hormone of love and responsible for the milk ejection reflex) – play an important role in how we feel emotionally... As breastfeeding ends, both prolactin and oxytocin levels will lower – and so may your mood and well-being. It may last a few days, or it may go on for longer. (Fieth 2020)

Thus no breastfeeding parent should be encouraged to stop

breastfeeding their babies unless they particularly wish to do so. If they do wish to stop, it is important to warn them that they may feel mixed feelings about it and may experience some low mood, often similar to that around menstruation.

PERSONAL STORY
Jennifer with Cherry and Alice

When I was going through the darkest time of my life after having the twins, even though I was constantly told I would feel better if I stopped breastfeeding to let other people 'take some of the load', I knew this wasn't going to help at all. I knew that continuing to do what brought me immense joy, and the only thing that was creating a bond between us, was going to be the single thing that kept us all together and me from jumping of that edge. I am so proud of myself for being so determined to feed, I feel I have shown the mental health care professionals that breastfeeding does in fact help and not hinder the mother's wellbeing. I even got a big applause when I was discharged from the mother and baby unit as they had never seen someone so determined and never learned so much about the importance of breastfeeding to the mother and the children.

Hannah with Josh and Tommy

For me, removing any expectation of getting anything else done apart from caring for the boys really helped me enjoy the early days. I had my babies in September and I remember thinking of Christmas as a milestone on the horizon, and to not worry about doing anything at all before then! With my husband's paternity leave largely used up while we were still in hospital, I had to get comfortable accepting help from others. My mum was amazing; she would let herself in while I was still in bed and do chores and hold the babies while I got showered. My mother-in-law also never came round without doing something helpful like hanging some washing or washing up. I found getting outside for walks in the fresh air really helped – the babies would sleep for longer in a moving pram, and I felt better for getting out. My main memory from the early days is camping out on the sofa under the tandem feeding pillow and eating dinner over the top of their heads while they cluster fed all evening. At the time it felt like it went on forever, but now I miss it!

Sarah with Lowri and Caelan

I sometimes find it useful to visualise breastfeeding (or even parenting) as a rollercoaster. Sometimes the train chugs slowly and noisily uphill, gears cranking, motors whirring, feeling like the little wheels will never reach the top because the train just can't do it. Then suddenly the carriages pop over the summit and whizz off, freewheeling down the track with lovely views and passengers squealing in delight.

Then the train plunges into a dark tunnel and you can't see the next bit of track or the way ahead. It always re-emerges into the daylight again though.

It's very literally a rollercoaster ride with high points, low points, and lots of chugging round the track – but the train does keep moving onwards.

Coping with older siblings

With a first baby (or babies), as a parent you can really concentrate on establishing breastfeeding, have a baby moon where you sit on the sofa all day having skin to skin, sleep when the baby sleeps and so on.

Having a set of twins or triplets as your second or later pregnancy often causes a lot of worry. Parents wonder how they will cope? They cannot sit around all day and feed. Older siblings still need attention, they need support with the transition to the new family dynamic and with the big feelings around being a sibling, and they need entertaining! Then there's the school or nursery run to do. Parents often feel totally torn between their older children and new babies' needs. Here are some suggestions of useful ideas to help.

- Get support! We are not supposed to parent alone. Have family around, have childcare for the older ones, partner or other helper can take over older siblings' bedtimes, friends

123

can be invited to come round for play dates and to cuddle a baby, perhaps the parents could employ a post-natal doula to help out, or see if there are any local parenting charities that can help. Some further education colleges teaching childcare courses also need placements for their students, who can be utilised as helpers.

- Go out! There may be a safe place locally where toddler can run free, maybe with the babies in the sling so the parent can more easily chase the older child. They can find activities for the older siblings where there are also comfortable sofas to feed. They could meet with other parents at groups who may be able to chase their toddler, or hold a baby while the parent does!

- A really useful tip can be to have a busy box at home, a box of toys that comes out when the babies are feeding. This is especially effective if the toys look like something they are not normally allowed! That makes it more exciting. With a small table and chair next to the sofa the toddler can do jigsaws, drawing, playdough, stickers, read books, and have snacks within easy reach, while the nursing parent is sitting feeding the babies right beside them.

- Although too much screen time is not ideal, it is incredibly useful to put on an older child's favourite programme, whether that be on the TV or hand held device, during feeds. Parents should try not to feel guilty about using screens. Once the babies are a bit less intense they can limit screen time again if necessary.

- Involving the older children in the care of the babies as much as possible helps them to feel involved. They can be asked to fetch nappies, fill the parent's water bottle, watch the babies for feeding cues, smell the babies' nappies for poo, fetch snacks, and pretend to feed their dolls/toys alongside the parent.

- Sometimes single feeding is easier when there are older siblings around. Parents can feed a baby just holding them with one hand, and can get up while breastfeeding to deal with the older one; they will soon become a pro at breastfeeding on the move. Of course, tandem feeding means that the feed is over more quickly so it depends on the parent's priorities. With a good supportive feeding cushion set up, parents can feed hands free so they can help with activities. There are pros and cons to both so it is just a matter of finding out what the parent finds easier and most convenient – and it doesn't have to be the same every time.

- Sleep whenever they can! The old adage 'sleep when your babies sleep' just is not possible with older siblings. If the older sibling is still having a nap, trying to coordinate the babies' nap time can be incredibly useful, although it is quite difficult to do this! If it does happen, parents should make sure they take advantage of it – perhaps by trying to get some sleep themselves, or they may prefer to just sit with a hot cup of tea in silence for a bit.

- Remember that toddlers and older children, although they still need their parents, are not reliant on them for everything. They can get their own snacks, for example. Setting up a place for them to help themselves to some healthy snacks can work well. Babies need their parents for everything. The older ones will actually adjust very quickly.

- If parents have places to be, the school run, nursery drop off, health appointments, toddler groups etc., then being super organised helps with getting to places on time. Repacking the changing bag whenever they get in means they can just pick it up on the way out. Trying to have places for coats, shoes, school bags, and other regularly needed equipment will help prevent the last minute search for stuff. Aiming to leave plenty of time to get anywhere is essential because it takes ten times longer to get out of the house than you think with multiple babies and older children in tow. Expect a last minute poo from at least one baby. Trying to feed the babies as the last thing before leaving means that hopefully they will not need feeding on the go. On the other hand, embrace that the babies may need feeding while out and about. Playground and waiting room feeds can work. If the parents are late for things, which will almost certainly happen at some point, it is totally fine to use the fact they have multiples as an excuse!

- Accepting that motherhood equals guilt is important. We feel guilty about everything, but it is ok to be just good enough. A perfect parent is not a thing! Providing siblings for an older child or children is something that the older ones are likely to value for their entire lives.

PERSONAL STORY
Catherine with Antigone and Hebe

When my twins were born their older siblings were six, four, and two. Life was already busy and the idea of adding two babies at once into the mix was pretty daunting. Of course, the elder two were already seasoned older siblings. I had always included them in looking after the next baby – helping to unfold nappies and standing on a stool to help during nappy changes, snuggling up on the sofa to read books together while I was feeding the baby, and so on. I prepared for the twins by getting a nice high up pram for them to sleep in downstairs – out of reach of big sisters who might not realise how much loving was too much for a tiny baby! – and modifying a full-size cot to fit onto the side of my bed to make night feeds easier.

When the twins were first born, life was very intense for a while. The older children still had school and pre-school to go to – the two-year-old turned two and a half two weeks after the twins were born, and was then able to go to pre-school two mornings a week so that I had a bit of time with just the babies. My lovely mother-in-law very kindly paid for us to have a cleaner, which was a massive help.

I switched to online shopping, and very quickly got the hang of carrying one or both babies in a stretchy or woven wrap. I did a lot of chores and bedtimes for the older three with one or both babies strapped to me. In the first few months I really didn't have time to stop and think, but it soon eased off a bit. The older ones loved having the twins to play with and the twins idolised their older brother and sisters, and we settled into our new normal.

Annie with Henry and Eadie (and William and Elizabeth)

Breastfeeding twins when you have a toddler or, in my case, two toddlers (who are also twins!) can be daunting, bringing lots of doubt as to how it can be at all possible to look after so many young people at once. It is absolutely possible! I had my second set of twins when my first set were just 16 months old. I exclusively breastfed them for the first six months, when I introduced solids. Here are some of my top tips on how to get through those first few weeks and months breastfeeding twins when you also have toddler(s).

I would focus on getting through that day. Not the week, not the month. I slowed it right down and just worked towards getting through it a day at a time.

There were some days where it felt really tough, but I believe bottle feeding would actually have made things more difficult. I used to sit on the floor and tandem feed the baby twins on my breastfeeding pillow, while reading stories or playing with Lego with the big twins. Bottle feeding would've been trickier as I wouldn't have had my hands free. I used to put the baby twins in a skin to skin top and quickly prep lunch while they breastfed snuggled in my t-shirt. I could take them all out for a walk and breastfeed the babies in the park without taking lots of extra things with me or worrying if I'd forgotten anything. At night time I didn't need to worry about the baby twins waking the big twins, as I would breastfeed them as soon as they woke instead of leaving them to cry and wake the house up if I had to go and prepare bottles. I kept reminding myself of the positives when it all got too much.

I tried to be organised. I put a basket of toys in each room for the big twins to play with. I would make sure there was a change of clothes and nappies in the main rooms we use in the house. It just made every day so much easier. On the days I didn't do this, I found myself scrambling around trying to find things in washing piles or at the bottom of toy boxes or looking all over for a pack of wipes. If I had things I needed to hand and I was busy feeding the little babies it meant I could quickly deal with what the big twins needed and keep some calmness in the house.

My motto was 'choose the easy options'! Yes, it would be lovely to get crafty with the toddlers, but in reality it would cause a huge amount of mess and stress. Easy options were painting my cupboard doors with a pot of water and clean paintbrushes. They had fun and there wasn't much mess. Invisible ink pens, magic water books, and bath/shower play with water toys were all my easy alternatives. I also love cooking, but my easy alternative was using my slow cooker. I got the satisfaction of everyone having a home-made nutritious meal together without having to spend hours cooking and have lots of mess to clean up. And now we are back enjoying lots of messy crafts with four toddlers!

Top Tips for Parents

Babies like to feed a lot. Eight feeds in 24 hours, three-hourly, is a minimum. Most prefer to feed more often.

Babies like to feed for all sorts of reasons, not just hunger and thirst, all are valid!

Offer a second go on the breast. Babies will trigger another let-down of milk and take some more. Encourage this if babies are a bit sleepy by waking them with a nappy change after the first go on the breast.

Try tandem feeding. You do not have to do it all the time, but it is very useful if both babies need to feed at the same time. Ask for support with this if you are struggling.

Responsive feeding is important, first to meet the needs of your babies, but also to ensure you make enough milk.

Babies should be doing at least six wet nappies and two good size poos in 24 hours.

Babies should be settled in someone's arms between feeds, except during cluster feeding periods.

Babies should be back to birth weight by three weeks at the latest, plotted on the growth chart from two weeks of age. They should then roughly be tracking this percentile line. We do not need them to go back up to the birth percentile.

Babies prefer to sleep on a human. It is normal for babies to wake immediately that you put them down. You are not spoiling them by cuddling them.

Prepare to do little else other than feed, cuddle, and change nappies in the first few weeks.

Invest in a sling – a stretchy wrap can be used for one or both babies in the early days. This means you can give the babies the security they need and have your hands free.

Line up lots of things to watch! And entertainment for older children.

Get help with all of the other things, housework, cooking, older siblings.

Try to get out for a walk every day, once you are physically able.

Visitors must do something useful in order to earn a cuddle. They can make their own tea and bring you food, as well as helping with household jobs.

Explore safe bed-sharing options. If you feel you are going to fall asleep with your babies it is far safer to do so in a well set up bed than anywhere else in your house.

Do not be afraid to ask for help and support from family and friends, and health care professionals and breastfeeding support. We are not designed to do this alone.

Pumping occasionally

Some parents like to express for the occasional bottle or if they have to leave their babies for some reason. Some like to express for a feed a day to get some sleep. Others may like to make a small stash in the freezer if they have something coming up in the future or just so they have it in emergencies.

It can be the case that to express the volume needed for a whole feed for both babies will take two or three pumping sessions. Particularly once the milk supply regulates to babies' needs, the pump is really just taking the leftovers. Expressing at a similar time each day can prime the breasts to make more milk at that time of day. Many parents find they will get a larger yield in the mornings than in the evenings. If the babies have a stretch of longer sleep sometimes this can be a good time to express.

A lot of parents worry about their milk supply if they are not getting much yield from their pumping sessions. The truth is, the volume they can get from pumping bears little resemblance to the amount of milk removed by a full term healthy baby who is latching on well at the breast. In general, babies who are feeding well can access the milk that the pump cannot extract.

One of the reasons for this is the hormonal response. Putting a pump to the chest elicits a weaker hormonal response than that elicited putting the baby to the chest. Let's face it, pumps do not naturally encourage the oxytocin to flow. It is very hard to bond with a bit of plastic that many feel is tying them down and taking them away from their baby. Remember, oxytocin is the hormone which triggers the milk ejection reflex, or let-down, and so is instrumental in delivering the milk to the baby, or to the pump. Oxytocin is produced when parents cuddle babies (especially in skin to skin contact), latch babies, hear them cry, smell their scent, or even just think about them. It is commonly known as the love hormone, and aids bonding.

The sucking mechanism of the pump does not work in the same way as a baby sucking on the breast. It is a man-made machine trying to emulate nature. Pumps rely on making a vacuum which draws out the milk. Babies also make a vacuum to draw out the milk, but it is paired with the baby's tongue and palate massaging the breast, and also they often use their hands to knead the breast, which increases the flow. In addition to this, some standard pumps are not very efficient and can only take the easy flowing milk at the start of the session.

The 'hands-on pumping' technique, the act of massaging and hand expressing before, during and after the pumping session, can help. Massaging increases oxytocin levels and helps to bring down the milk so it can be removed by the pump more easily. Research shows this technique can increase yield by up to 48%. Having the babies close by, looking at photos or videos of the babies, or smelling their scent on their clothes if they have to be separated encourages the oxytocin to flow.

There is no need to have a stash of milk, but if the parent wishes to make one they can just pump whenever they get the chance. Maybe once a day, or perhaps a couple of times a week. If adding freshly expressed milk to some which has been refrigerated from a previous pumping session, the new milk must be chilled to the same temperature as the stored milk before mixing, so as not to add warm milk to cold. The milk can then be stored in the freezer for future use, labelled with the date of the earliest expressing session. However, as milk must be discarded once the baby's saliva has touched the vessel, storing in large quantities can risk throwing away unwanted milk. It is often better to store in smaller volumes because of this.

Many parents think they would like to express for a bottle so they can have a break from the babies, but in reality finding time to express and adding in the additional washing up, sterilising, and preparation, they often decide it is easier just to breastfeed and not worry about bottles. It is really up to the parent to decide if the hassle of pumping is worth the break they will get later.

Milk storage

There are varying guidelines available as to how long expressed human milk can be stored in different temperature and scenarios. This information and table is from the Centers for Disease Control and Prevention (the national public health agency of the United States).

Proper storage and preparation of breast milk

	Counter top 25°C or cooler	Refrigerator 4°C	Freezer -18°C
Freshly expressed milk	Up to 4 hours	Up to 4 days	Within 6 months best, up to 12 months is acceptable
Defrosted milk	1–2 hours	Up to 1 day	Do not refreeze human milk
Leftover from feeding baby	Use within 2 hours after baby has finished feeding		

Source: Centers for Disease Control and Prevention (2021)

Expressed milk can be used immediately or stored in the fridge or freezer. It should always be stored in breast milk storage bags or food grade containers, glass or non-bisphenol A (BPA) plastic. It should be clearly labelled with the date it was expressed. It must not be stored in the door of the fridge, as the temperature is less stable. If transporting expressed milk, a cool bag with ice blocks may be used for up to 24 hours.

Defrosting frozen milk is best done in the refrigerator overnight or, if it is needed quickly, stand in warm water or run under warm running water. Never defrost milk in the microwave as it can destroy nutrients and create hot spots (Centers for Disease Control and Prevention 2021).

Pump parts should be washed after each use in hot soapy water or dishwasher if appropriate (check manufacturer's guidelines) and air dry. Pump cleaning equipment (bottle brush and basin) should also be cleaned regularly. For extra protection you may wish to sterilise pump parts once a day, though this may not be necessary for older, healthy babies if pump parts are cleaned thoroughly (Centers for Disease Control and Prevention 2020).

Exclusive pumping

Some parents may decide to continue to pump for their babies and not introduce the breast after a NICU journey. Or perhaps their babies never latch and so they make the decision to express and give their milk to their babies via another method. Some may choose to pump for all sorts of other personal reasons.

Exclusively pumping, or pumping for the majority of a baby's feeds, is hard work and is by far the most difficult and time consuming way to feed babies. However, it is possible, and a choice some parents make. Once milk supply is established, the parent can work out how many pumping sessions in 24 hours they will need to do in order to maintain production. This is very individual and is influenced by the parent's natural milk storage capacity, as well as how they respond to the pump. Some parents with a large storage capacity may find they can meet their baby's intake with fewer pumping sessions, while others may need to pump far more frequently to maintain production. Normally most parents start by pumping around 8 times in 24 hours, then once they are making enough milk for their babies they can experiment with stopping one pumping session and see if yield continues. They may also need to adjust the timings of the other sessions.

Nancy Mohrbacher states in her blog 'The "magic number" and long-term milk production':

> The 'magic number.' This refers to the number of times each day a mother's breasts need to be well drained of milk to keep her milk production stable. Due to differences in breast storage capacity, some mothers' 'magic number' may be as few as 4–5 or as many as 9–10. But when a mother's total number of breast drainings (breastfeedings plus milk expressions) dips below her 'magic number,' her milk production slows. (Mohrbacher 2010)

If production is maintained then they can continue with fewer expressions. If production drops then they may have to reinstate that pumping session. If production continues with one fewer pumping session, they may be able to cut out another and assess the outcome.

For those who manage with less frequent pumping sessions, they will often find this journey much easier than those who need to pump more frequently. Those that need to pump more frequently may end up pumping more often than their babies feed, which is challenging, especially once the babies begin to sleep for a longer stretch. It is important to support each individual family and adjust to their particular situation.

PERSONAL STORY
Laura with Florence and Ada

After a relatively stress free pregnancy I went for my 36 week scan and found that Twin One had turned breech, and I had developed severe pre-eclampsia, so I was to have a section in two days. During the section the girls were born safely but then things got tense and I had a massive bleed and became very ill. I had 24/7 nursing care and got told my kidneys had gone into failure and I might have to be ventilated!

Through all this the midwives knew that I wanted to breastfeed, and were great at manually expressing colostrum (at a time when I couldn't do anything for my girls this was at least something I was doing for them!). Due to concerns with my kidneys, my fluid intake and output was monitored really carefully and it was suggested I pump rather than directly breastfeed for a couple of days. I did this and got into such a good routine with it that I actually then had no inclination to get them to latch (despite midwives and HV offering). We were in a good routine and it was working so I stuck at it. When I was discharged I hired the pump I had been using at the hospital as I had no idea how long I would be pumping for and didn't want to fork out for one and then not end up using it for long.

After two weeks of formula top ups we dropped the formula and all feeds were expressed breast milk. I continued pumping six times a day/night and ended up with so much that I needed to buy a new freezer to store it in! I obviously was lucky and had a naturally good supply. I did this for seven months, at which point I started to struggle to find the time to express so often with two active seven-month-olds (and getting up to express in the night while the girls continued to sleep was a killer!) so, with advice and support from the Breastfeeding Twins and Triplets UK Facebook group, I gradually weaned off pumping, used my massive frozen stocks and when they ran out went onto formula. It was nothing like the journey I thought I would have, and during my pregnancy I never even knew exclusively expressing was an option, but although it had it challenges it really worked for us!

Combination feeding

There is little evidence regarding making enough milk for two or three babies. Milk supply works on a demand and supply basis – having two or three babies coming to the breast means the breasts are stimulated two or three times more than those feeding a singleton, so they should produce two or three times the milk (Saint, Maggiore & Hartmann 1986).

When I speak to expectant multiple parents, many assume that they will have to combination feed. Our society, friends, family, and health professionals all believe it is difficult, even impossible, to make enough milk for more than one baby. However, with good breastfeeding support and frequent and efficient feeds, most find they can make enough milk for their twin or triplet babies. I usually suggest giving breastfeeding a really good go to start with as it is far easier to move from breastfeeding to formula than it is from formula to breastfeeding.

Around 40% of twin babies and nearly all triplet and higher order multiples are born premature or unwell and have to go to the neonatal unit (Twins Trust 2020). In this situation the breastfeeding journey is started via expressing colostrum and breast milk, and feeding via a tube. Frequent pumping with a hospital grade double pump will give the best chance of establishing a copious supply (Hill *et al.* 2005) but, as the babies grow and become more efficient feeders, milk supply becomes easier to establish by feeding directly. There seems to be little research into whether there is a window of opportunity to establish a full milk supply. It is certainly possible to increase milk volumes several months into breastfeeding.

The majority of twins are born around 36 to 37 weeks gestation. This can mean they struggle initially as, even though a twin pregnancy is deemed as 'full term' at 37 weeks, the babies are not full term babies! They can be quite small, sleepy, and inefficient on the breast to begin with (Ayton *et al.* 2012). These babies sometimes need topping up with expressed milk or formula after a feed to start with, as discussed in Chapter 4. Parents start by breastfeeding the babies, topping up with expressed if they have it, or formula if they don't, by cup, syringe, or bottle, and then double pumping with a hospital grade pump. They find they are combination feeding even if it was never their plan to do so. As the babies approach 40 week gestation, they often start feeding more effectively and top ups can be gradually phased out, though some parents will choose to continue combination feeding as they have got used to it by this point.

Multiples that are born closer to full term are likely to struggle less with breastfeeding, and so as long as the parent is supported to feed frequently with optimum positioning and attachment, the breasts should be stimulated sufficiently to make enough milk for more than one baby. Tandem feeding can often help make feeding more efficient and will help the parents cope with fussy behaviour and cluster feeding, and there may well be no need for combination feeding.

There may be a point where the family think they are at maximum capacity for breastfeeding and milk production, whether this is at some point during the journey of establishing supply, or after a full supply has been established. This can occasionally be because of physiological reasons for not being able to produce enough milk (this is actually pretty rare), a difficult start with breastfeeding where milk supply was never fully established, or for other reasons – for example to do with mental health.

Combination feeding can be a good option for these families – it is so important to value every drop of breast milk each baby receives. Formula can be a useful tool to prolong the breastfeeding relationship if used in a considered way.

Many families start by breastfeeding and then topping up with formula, however this is not really something that can be kept up long term. Feeding both breast and bottle every feed can be too much work, especially once a co-parent has gone back to work. If there are physiological reasons for low supply, using a supplemental nursing system can be a great option. The babies can be topped up at the breast and so the breastfeeding relationship is protected and milk supply will be maximised.

Many families prefer to give one or two set bottle feeds of formula a day and breastfeed responsively in between. This pattern is often suggested when the babies are struggling with weight gain, and some families choose to keep it long term. It is protective of breastfeeding as long as the babies are being breastfed responsively the rest of the time, and the parents don't fall into the 'top up trap' when babies are fussy or feeding more frequently. The top up trap is the name used to refer to the process where as babies need more milk, more formula is offered, and so babies come to the breast less. This then means less milk is produced by the breast, which then means more formula is needed, and the cycle repeats until the babies begin to refuse the breast because of low milk supply. So breastfeeding responsively in between set bottle feeds (with both fixed time and fixed milk volumes) prevents this from happening. If the bottle feed can be given by someone other than the breastfeeding parent, this can be a good way of having a break, getting more sleep, or spending more time with older children.

For triplet families, as well as the twin related scenarios discussed above, there is also the issue that there are more babies than breasts! Various patterns of breastfeeding, expressing, and formula feeding can be adopted, as discussed in the Triplets box in Chapter 5. Although it is entirely possible to exclusively feed triplets directly at the breast, for many triplet families a combination of breast and bottle feeding works for them – and of course the combination of breast, bottles of expressed breast milk, and formula bottles can change as time passes, according to the family's needs at the time. For higher order multiples, similar patterns can be adopted.

PERSONAL STORIES
Kristy with Carwyn and Addison

When I first tried breastfeeding I found it really difficult. I didn't get much support in the hospital and I was by myself as a new mom of twins. They had a lot of formula to start with, and I'd try to breastfeed each day but found it painful and hard. I kept persisting and received support when I left hospital from my health visitor and later an independent consultant. The kindest thing they said was to not look at formula as something stopping me breastfeeding but as an aid to *keep* me breastfeeding as it took the pressure off worrying about whether they were getting anything, and in the early days when breastfeeding was really painful I didn't feel like I had to put myself through it.

With support and practice, and the help of formula at certain times, I've managed to breastfeed and am still breastfeeding now at 14 months! I plan to keep feeding until they're two – if I hadn't used combination feeding in the early days I'm not sure I would have reached this goal. Ultimately they've got more breast milk from me, and for a longer period of time. I love breastfeeding now! And I think it's because I didn't have any undue pressure put on me.

Yasmin with Ophelia and Hector

As soon as we found out we were having twins everyone I knew wanted to know how I was going to feed them, and when I said breastfeeding they looked horrified and said I would never manage it! I managed to exclusively breastfeed the twins until six weeks, at that point I made the decision to combi feed. The twins started having a bottle of formula at 7pm and eventually after a few more weeks they had a bottle of formula at 7am as well. I never got on with expressing with my two previous singletons, so I knew this wasn't something I wanted to do. I also knew that wanting to have a break of an evening, and for someone else to be able to feed them, was important. The babies both love having a bottle now, but equally still love breastfeeding. When it comes to feeding lots of people like to tell you what's best, but only you will know what's best for you and your babies.

Ruth with Samuel and Naomi

I have insufficient glandular tissue and never made a full milk supply for my two singletons. Before they were born, one of my apprehensions about breastfeeding twins was the logistics of feeding both together or one after the other, and also how that would work with our set up with the supplemental nursing system (SNS).

I have been so pleased with my secondhand tandem feeding pillow. It fits my body shape and size brilliantly, and is so comfortable for the three of us. I don't tandem feed all the time, less so when I have help to entertain the other one, and often even if both are on the pillow with me they're not necessarily both feeding simultaneously, sometimes I'm just holding the non-feeding one sat up next to me. I'm also really pleased with how our homemade supplemental nursing systems have worked this time. Our version is basically an ordinary baby bottle with a thin (size French 4) NG tube pushed through the teat. I find this system easier to clean and sterilise than the branded one, and the flow seems easier to regulate. I can rest the bottle on the tandem pillow or hold it in my hand when single feeding.

It's such a good feeling to be able to say that the twins have been fed exclusively at the breast for six months! They haven't had a single bottle in that time, and I don't intend that they will ever need one now. Of course they have had formula to top up my supply, but it's all been consumed via the SNS. This means they have maximised the amount of milk they've got from me, and we've been able to enjoy the benefits of a breastfeeding relationship that go beyond the milk. I know that for twins we are blessed to be in this situation. It's not unusual for twins to be born early and therefore struggle to feed at the breast for days, weeks or months. Despite my chronic low supply, we've had it quite easy in this respect. Strangely I don't feel that unusual in the twin breastfeeding world compared to in the singleton breastfeeding world. I think it's because lots of twins end up being mixed fed breast milk and formula at some point, either short or long term. It took me to have twins to feel like I belong!

Chapter 8

Common Problems

It is important to remember that multiple birth babies are just babies, and multiple birth parents are just parents. So the families are susceptible to all the same feeding issues as any other family. In some instances, because of the increased volume of milk production and early delivery, they can be slightly more susceptible to certain breastfeeding difficulties. If the parents are already overwhelmed with having to cope with more than one baby, sometimes these difficulties, often fairly simple to improve, can tip them over the edge and result in parents stopping breastfeeding earlier than they had hoped. However, many families manage to push through all sorts of problems and continue to meet or exceed their goals. The key is to be prepared in advance and to access support early!

Not latching

It is fairly common for new babies to refuse to latch or not be able to latch in the early days. There can be all sorts of causes: traumatic birth, drugs in labour, early birth, sleepy babies, small babies, small mouths, tongue tie, flat or inverted nipples, large breasts or nipples. Sometimes it is all of the twins or triplets who are struggling. Sometimes it is just one.

If this is happening it is important to remember that with support the majority of babies do eventually latch on and breastfeed. Having plenty of skin to skin time will help baby's natural instincts to kick in, and it may be that once baby has woken up a bit they are able to latch quite easily. Give the baby as much opportunity as possible.

Obviously babies that are not latching still need to be fed! Parents can be encouraged to hand express colostrum and this can be given to the baby by syringe, teaspoon, or cup at regular intervals. Sometimes giving the baby some expressed colostrum will give them the energy they need to latch on and breastfeed. If the baby continues not to latch as milk comes in, then parents can move onto a hospital grade pump and express milk for the baby. As with colostrum, this milk can be given by syringe, teaspoon, cup, or bottle. It is important to be aware that if a bottle is introduced it is imperative to pace the feed, as the baby may be even less likely to latch if they get used to a fast flow of milk from a bottle.

Frequent expressing will help establish and protect the parent's milk production while they are waiting for their baby to be able to breastfeed. If parents can establish a good supply then when baby is able to breastfeed directly the milk will be there for them.

If the baby continues to refuse the breast, parents can find their local breastfeeding support. Sometimes it is a matter of improving latching technique, which will get babies feeding. Sometimes breast compressions will help a baby begin to take milk from the breast as this makes the milk flow. Sometimes an oral assessment will find a restricted tongue or high palate, or even a missed cleft, in which case baby may need to be referred for other treatment options.

A baby who has had lots of bottles may sometimes need to be coaxed onto the breast with use of a nipple shield. The silicone shield makes the breast feel more like a bottle teat, and will often trigger baby's suck reflex more effectively if they have been used to the firmer stimulus of the bottle teat.

Sometimes babies may be coaxed onto the breast when they are incredibly calm and not hungry. Lots of skin to skin will get the oxytocin flowing, which helps to calm the baby and also to boost milk supply. Offering the breast just as baby is stirring from a nap – at the earliest feeding cues – means they are more likely to latch than if they are starving hungry and screaming. Offering a small bottle feed first and then offering the breast for comfort afterwards can do the trick. Sharing a bath with baby can make them so chilled that they latch.

One baby not latching

If one twin is breastfeeding directly and the other is not latching this can cause all sorts of mixed emotions. Guilt is often the main one, as the breastfed baby will automatically get more cuddles and more connection through feeding. Parents can find it more difficult to bond with the bottle fed baby. Many will pump their milk for the bottle fed baby so at least they can feel like they are getting the same health benefits of human milk, even if they cannot feed directly.

Sometimes one baby may be unwell and not be able to feed. In some sets of twins or triplets, health conditions, illness, need for surgery etc., can all mean that one of the babies is not able to directly breastfeed. One baby may have to stay in hospital long term. This is an incredibly difficult situation, but hospitals can ease pressure on parents by allowing the well baby into the hospital with the breast-feeding parent, so they can continue to establish their breastfeeding relationship while also caring for the unwell baby. Once the unwell baby has recovered and is able to begin to feed, breastfeeding can be introduced. Many assume that if babies are not breastfed from the beginning they will not be able to start, but this is actually not the case at all.

The important thing in this situation is to keep trying. After a few weeks they may not want to try latching every feed, or even every day, as the refusal can be stressful to deal with. But giving a go now and then to see what happens can have surprising results! Sometimes babies will start to latch after a tongue tie division, or just after they have grown a bit bigger. It is even sometimes possible to start breastfeeding directly after cleft surgery, despite the baby often being many months old. In the Breastfeeding Twins and Triplets UK Facebook group we have seen babies suddenly start latching at four, five, or six months, when they have never breastfed before. The milk production is there because the parents have been pumping or breastfeeding the other baby, so if babies do latch at this point they will get milk.

Sadly, sometimes nothing works. In this case parents may make the decision to pump for one baby and breastfeed the other. There are a few hacks to make this easier. Parents can pump from the other side while the baby is breastfeeding, which not only saves doing the pumping after the feed, but also the feeding baby stimulates the hormones so the parent can express more milk in less time. Some will also manage to bottle feed the other baby at the same time with the help of a supportive feeding cushion and a hands free pumping bra.

PERSONAL STORY
Kayleigh with Daisy and Rose

At 19 weeks pregnant I found out that one of my twins had a unilateral cleft lip and more than likely cleft palate, meaning her chances of latching to feed would be very small. When she was born it was very obvious she had palate involvement too. This is where my pumping journey began for Rose. I did grieve that I wouldn't be able to feed her direct and there were certainly lots of tears! But I was also very happy to have two healthy baby girls and the cleft lip was an isolated occurrence, as it was suggested during the pregnancy that there could have been more health issues.

I knew I wanted to breastfeed Daisy as I had breastfed my first little girl for 16 months. But I was so torn on feeding one and not the other. This made me determined to try and express for Rose. Those first six weeks of pumping three-hourly, then bottle feeding her and breastfeeding on top were so difficult. I am currently eight and half months into expressing and feeding and have no intentions of stopping. I am so proud I managed to keep up the expressing for Rose as health professionals didn't seem to think it would be manageable! The Facebook support I have received from other twin mums has been wonderful, with so many inspirational women.

Amy with Alison and Toby

I was very lucky as the bigger twin (the girl) came out and latched almost immediately. But my boy had a bowel condition and had to go to the neonatal unit. I co-slept with my girl in the hospital from birth. Even the breastfeeding team in the NNU said she breastfed like a YouTube star, and after my first baby (who stank at breastfeeding!) this was a joy to behold. She fed fast and efficiently and then slept the day away next to her brother.

The support in the NNU was exceptional, but they were very pro babies getting breast milk but at the same time very anti breastfeeding, as they said there was no way to monitor what baby got during a breastfeed. They were set against it from the start, so pumping was something I did after each feed regardless of how much I got. Not comfortable to pump and feed at same time in hospital due to the chairs, I would feed her, pop her down, then pump. I managed all this eight times in 24 hours, and I was so exhausted. I was given a galactagogue to help production – it worked well, and I was soon pumping 700–800ml per day on top of what my girl was taking directly.

One day I could go no further emotionally, it was two months in, I needed to breastfeed him. After much tears and wrangling I was allowed. That day I left him in a deep milk slumber. I felt like I had actually done something for him for the first time in two months. They talk about milk in terms of weight gain but there is no acknowledgement of the mothers' need to feed their babies through something other than a tube.

Sore or cracked nipples, causes

Many people will experience sore or cracked nipples. It is important to remember that pain throughout the feed is not normal and indicates there is something wrong. Sometimes parents will be told that pain is normal in the first few weeks, but this is not true. There is sometimes some initial latching pain which may last for a few seconds just as baby is attaching to the breast, but the majority of the feed should be comfortable.

The most common cause of pain when breastfeeding is a shallow latch. If the baby is not getting a large mouthful of breast tissue, the nipple does not go back far enough into the roof of the mouth and rubs on the hard palate. After feeds the nipple often looks compressed and lipstick shaped, with a ridge. If this continues, the ridge can crack and bleed, and bacterial or yeast infection can get into the crack.

A shallow latch can also cause vasospasm, causing it to look blanched and be painful after the feed, or milk blisters (also known as blebs). These present as a small white dot on the surface of the nipple, often more visible just after a feed. A bleb is basically a blocked nipple pore, and occurs when a tiny bit of skin grows over the opening. Milk can back up behind it, and causes pain at the site and also pain further into the breast as the milk backs up in the ducts. Clearing the blockage should resolve the pain. Look for a small white, clear, or yellow dot on the nipple. They can be caused by friction from a shallow latch or similar causes to blocked ducts (see next section). Apply moist heat prior to breastfeeding, clear the skin away gently with a clean finger nail or rub with a flannel, and breastfeed or pump to help move the blockage. They can be quite persistent and are often quite painful.

If the parent has sought expert breastfeeding support and the symptoms continue, tongue tie should be ruled out. A tongue tie is when the frenulum (a strip of tissue which is below the tongue and part of normal anatomy) is restricted, meaning that the tongue cannot move as it should. A tongue tie practitioner or IBCLC can perform an oral assessment checking tongue function and movement, and a feeding assessment to see how baby is transferring milk. If a restriction is found then referral to a tongue tie practitioner for division should help the situation.

Vasospasm may be caused by a shallow latch or a tongue tie. A vasospasm is a constriction of the blood vessels and causes a burning, stabbing pain. Nipples look blanched after a feed, and can be very painful. The cold often makes it worse, and some people find that pocket hand warmers to pop on after feeds can make a big difference to managing symptoms. Support with positioning and attachment will help. Keeping the breast warm and gentle massage can help alleviate the pain. The parent may know already that they suffer from Raynaud's syndrome – which is a disorder affecting the tiny blood vessels in the extremities and thus reducing blood flow. Warmth and sometimes medication can help if this is the cause.

Thrush, a yeast infection, can also cause sore nipples. It can present as a reddening of the nipple (more difficult to see on darker skin tones), and a loss of colour in the areola. It often makes the skin of the areola look shiny, and it tends to present in both breasts as it is very contagious. The babies are likely to also have symptoms: creamy white patches on the tongue, roof of the mouth, gums, and inside the cheeks and it can cause unsettled feeds as it is uncomfortable for baby. Treatment should be given to the breastfeeding parent and all babies, along with information about good hygiene.

Blocked ducts

The ducts in the breast are very fine and can block quite easily, either due to inflammation in the surrounding tissue or thickened milk, or both at once. The parent may feel a tender lump, and the skin around may look red and feel warm (difficult to see in darker skin tones). The inflammation caused by the blockage can then cause blockages in the surrounding ducts, leading to a larger painful area, like a traffic jam! Blockages can be caused by poor milk draining, perhaps by a poor latch, or something like a tight bra, car seatbelt, bag strap, or sling. Breast surgery or scar tissue can also cause blockages.

Treatment

- Continue to feed frequently with a deep latch.

- Baby should finish the breast, watch for them to move into their light fluttery sucking.

- Treat the inflammation with a cold compress.

- If the milk is flowing use some gentle breast compressions on the sections of the breast that may feel full.

- Gentle lymphatic massage can be used from nipple to armpit, with a similar amount of pressure as would be used applying lotion. This can be especially useful if the milk is backing up behind the blockage, or for swelling. Excess milk and fluid will drain from the lymph glands in the armpit. Firm massage should be avoided as it can damage the delicate ductal structure inside the breast and increase inflammation.

- The blockage should feel softer after feeds but may 'refill' in the lead up to the next feed. Gradually over a couple of days it should get better. If the blocked duct does not clear within a week or so the GP should refer to the breast clinic to check for other causes.

Mastitis

Mastitis is an inflammation of the breast usually caused by obstruction or infection. It may come on abruptly, and usually affects only one breast.

Symptoms may include

- A hard lump or wedge-shaped area of engorgement that may feel tender, hot, swollen or look reddened. On black and brown skin redness is less visible.

- The area may feel hot and tender or even quite painful.

- There may be red streaks extending outward from the affected area, again if it is visible.

- Fever, chills, flu-like aching, and feeling unwell.

- Milk may take on a saltier taste – some babies may refuse the breast due to this temporary change.

Treatment

- Take pain relief if necessary, paracetamol and ibuprofen are safe to take when breastfeeding as long as the parent is usually ok to take them. Ibuprofen also helps relieve swelling, which is very useful.

- Continue to feed frequently with a deep latch. Try a variety of positions. Some people find dangle feeding can help massively – with the parent on all fours and baby lying on their back looking up at the breast.

- Sometimes feeding seems too painful to manage but the milk still needs to be removed from the breast, so in this situation the parent should pump.

- As with any blocked duct, gentle lymphatic massage can be used from nipple to armpit, with a similar amount of pressure as would be used applying lotion. This can be especially useful if the milk is backing up behind the blockage, or for swelling. Excess milk and fluid will drain from the lymph glands in the armpit. Firm massage should be avoided as it can damage the delicate ductal structure inside the breast and increase inflammation.

- A warm compress before and during the feed can help the milk flow.

- Use a cold compress between feeds to reduce inflammation.

- Rest (not easy with two or three babies!).

- Drink plenty of fluids and make sure to have adequate nutrition.

- If there is no improvement within 12–24 hours go to the GP for some antibiotics.

Recurrent mastitis

If recurrent bouts of mastitis occur, it is important to identify any underlying causes. Sometimes the original course of antibiotics was not enough, or it may have been the incorrect antibiotic for the infection, and so the same infection increases again. Milk transfer should be assessed, and oral assessment performed to ensure baby has no tongue tie or other oral cavity issues that may prevent good breast drainage. Parents may have underlying health conditions making them more prone to infection. Sometimes breast cancer can present as recurrent mastitis.

Low supply

First it's really important to work out whether there is in fact low supply, or whether there has been a misunderstanding of normal baby behaviour. Many new parents are shocked by how frequently a baby will want to feed, and that babies are often unsettled for long periods, that they wake at night frequently and display cluster feeding behaviour. When there is more than one baby this makes it all worse of course! However, if the babies are feeding frequently, waking themselves for feeds, are generally settled in somebody's arms in between feeds (for the majority of the time – some cluster feeding and fussy periods are normal), they have lots of wet and dirty nappies, and weight gain is good, it is very likely that milk supply is just fine. Parents may worry that they amount they can pump is not what the baby takes from the bottle, but even hospital grade pumps are not as efficient as babies, so the amount a parent can get when pumping is no indication of what the babies take when they are feeding.

However, a small percentage of people may not be able to make a full milk supply. There are many reasons for low supply. Inefficient or infrequent removal of the milk is the most likely cause of low supply, and can usually be overcome with good support and information. There are also some pre-existing medical conditions which can cause a parent to struggle to make a full supply. There is no research as to the percentage of lactating people that would be able to make a full milk supply for twins or triplets, however there are many studies into singleton breastfeeding dyads which have found a range from 1–5% who are unable to make a full supply for one baby.

Poor breastfeeding management in the early days is one of the biggest risk factors for low supply. As mentioned earlier in the book, multiple birth parents have increased risk of inefficient removal of milk due to early or premature birth.

Risk factors for establishing supply include being separated from the babies after birth without sufficient hand expression and pumping, babies not feeding frequently due to being early term and sleepy, strict routines being suggested in order to cope with multiples, and topping up with formula without also pumping – which means the breasts do not get the message to make enough milk.

Supplemental feeds of formula lead to the babies spending less time at the breast. If formula is indicated as necessary then it is imperative that hand expressing or pumping to compensate for the babies not taking the milk is encouraged. Otherwise, as the babies feed less at the breast, more formula will be needed, eventually often leading to breast refusal. This is the 'top up trap', as discussed in the combination feeding section in Chapter 7.

Baby's breastfeeding skills can have an impact on low supply. Early babies are at greater risk of being inefficient at the breast, as we discussed earlier in the book. If they are not able to take enough milk to meet their needs, the breasts will not make that additional milk which is needed. There are also anatomical issues with the palate, jaw, and tongue that can have an impact on the efficiency of the feed.

The parent's anatomy may also have an impact on the baby's breastfeeding efficiency. Flat or inverted nipples, very large or long nipples, and very large breasts can make attachment onto the breast more challenging.

Mammary hypoplasia or insufficient glandular tissue (IGT) can mean that the parent does not have enough of the milk making tissue within their breasts. Indicators that this may be an issue can be hormonal issues, very small widely spaced or tubular shaped breasts, one breast is very much smaller than the other, or if there were no breast changes in pregnancy or no feeling of fullness after birth. The actual amount of milk parents are able to make with these conditions varies from a good amount to nearly nothing, so it is incredibly important to get breastfeeding off to a good start if any issues are suspected. It is sometimes the case that with each subsequent pregnancy a parent with IGT is able to make a slightly larger supply than they had previously.

Breast surgery has the potential to damage nerves and ducts and compromise glandular tissue. This includes breast reduction, breast implants, lumpectomy, abscess drainage, and past trauma to the chest, including chest drains, burns, radiation, or infections. Some types of surgery cause more damage than others but until a parent tries they will not know how much difference it has made.

Hormonal imbalance or need for fertility treatment can cause issues with milk production or the milk ejection reflex. These include polycystic ovary syndrome (PCOS), thyroid issues, diabetes, lutein cysts, low prolactin levels, and infertility. And, of course, pregnancy!

Some medications and herbs can interfere with milk production. Hormonal birth control, some birth related drugs, some decongestants, herbs such as sage, parsley, and mint if taken in excess, low iron levels, and excess alcohol and smoking can all have an impact.

If a parent has low supply then finding expert breastfeeding support is invaluable. Good positioning and attachment and a feeding plan tailored to the specific needs of the family will maximise the individual milk making potential of each parent.

Supplementing the babies at the breast with a supplemental nursing system (either homemade with a French 5 or 6 feeding tube and a bottle for each baby, or a shop bought one), can help maximise supply and protect breastfeeding, while ensuring the babies get enough milk. It protects against bottle preference, keeps babies interested in breastfeeding as it increases the flow of the milk, means the babies are also stimulating the breast during the top up which helps to increase milk supply, and means there is no need to give a separate feed for supplementary milk.

Engorgement and oversupply

Many parents, even of twins and triplets, find they make a bit too much milk in the first few weeks after their babies are born, or after starting their journey by pumping for babies in the neonatal unit. It sounds like a good thing but actually can be quite difficult to manage. It can cause babies to be very fussy on the breast, and windy and unsettled after feeding. It can also mean that the breastfeeding parent can find they need to continue to pump for comfort even once the babies are breastfeeding directly.

It is very common to have a bit of an oversupply when milk first comes in around day 2–5. Breasts may feel hard, tender, and engorged, and the babies may struggle to latch onto the swollen breast. It can make the parent more susceptible to blocked ducts and mastitis. When the babies latch the milk may come out so fast that the baby splutters and coughs and comes off the breast. This can cause the baby to be windy and unsettled as they swallow air when they cough and splutter. Sometimes it can cause breast refusal.

If the parent has been pumping and storing a lot of extra milk, they will need to cut down very gradually to reduce the oversupply. They should aim to decrease the total 24-hour volume a little every day. They can do this by pumping for a bit less time at each pumping session, or cut one pumping session out completely. In order for breasts to make less milk, some needs to be left in the breast and the breast needs to feel full – that way the feedback mechanism telling the body it is making too much milk will work. However, if they cut back too quickly it can cause severe engorgement and increase the likelihood of developing mastitis.

If oversupply continues to be a problem after all the above have been tried, it may be appropriate to use some herbs or medication to suppress lactation a little. But they should be used with caution to ensure supply is not reduced too much. Cabbage leaves, sage, or pseudoephedrine, usually found in decongestants, have all been used to reduce supply.

Top Tips for Parents

Breastfeed babies frequently. If breasts are left for a long time without milk being removed it will make the engorgement and fast flow worse.

Ensure babies have a deep latch. If they are latched on well, they will be able to deal with the flow much better.

Try feeding babies in a more upright position. They should be able to cope with the flow much more easily if their heads are higher than their hips.

Lean back when feeding. Gravity actually slows the flow down and makes it easier to feed.

If the babies come off when the let-down happens, let the milk spray into a muslin cloth. Once it settles the babies can re-latch. The flow should have subsided a little. Placing a flat hand over the nipple and pressing into the breast can help stop the squirt!

Hand express a little before the start the feed to trigger the let-down reflex. But be careful not to overstimulate supply!

If feeling uncomfortable it is important to try not to succumb to pumping as this will increase your milk supply and make the situation worse.

If your breasts are too hard and swollen for baby to latch easily then try reverse pressure softening: place fingers around the nipple and press into the breast and hold. This will help move the fluid back up into the breast and soften the areola, making it easier to latch.

Gentle sweeping massage from nipple up into the armpit helps. This is known as therapeutic breast massage or lymphatic drainage.

A cold compress between feeds can relieve swelling and a warm compress just before the feed can help the milk flow.

It is safe to take paracetamol and ibuprofen and breastfeed, as long as you are usually safe to take them. Ibuprofen also helps reduce inflammation.

After a few days or weeks most people find oversupply settles and milk production regulates to match what the babies are taking.

Assigning a breast to each baby may speed up the process of supply regulating to meet the babies' needs.

Reflux

Posseting some milk after each feed is completely normal and no treatment is needed. However, if they baby is bringing up large volumes and this is causing some weight gain issues, or if baby is distressed for the majority of the day (not just evening fussiness or a temporary growth spurt type behaviour) then there are some things that may help.

For reflux type symptoms investigations should be as follows:

- Face to face breastfeeding support. An improved latch often improves symptoms.

- Feed in an upright position. Koala hold or laid back works well. If the parent finds these difficult then ensure baby's head is higher than their hips in cradle/rugby hold.

- Keep the babies in an upright position after feeds. Of course this is more difficult with two babies. A sling can be a massive help!

- Feed frequently. Large infrequent feeds, especially by bottle, make symptoms worse.

- Use the paced bottle feeding technique if using bottles. Pacing the feed will lessen the risk of overfeeding which can make reflux symptoms worse. Babies will also take in less air if the bottle is paced.

- Cow's milk protein allergy (CMPA investigation): Does baby have any other symptoms of allergy? CMPA is one of the more common causes of reflux symptoms. If an allergy is suspected the breastfeeding parent can eliminate dairy from their diet and continue to breastfeed. After a few days symptoms should begin to improve, although it can take a few weeks for baby's gut to heal completely. Many CMPA babies are also allergic to soy so this may also need to be avoided by the parent.

- Tongue tie assessment. A tongue tie practitioner or IBCLC can do an oral assessment and assess tongue function. If a restriction is found a tongue tie division can improve reflux symptoms.

- Investigate different medications.

Too frequently health care professionals jump straight to medication without looking at the rest of the picture.

Breast refusal and nursing strikes

Sometimes babies become fussy on the breast or refuse to latch completely. This can be because the baby is receiving lots of bottles, or it can be developmental – it is quite commonly found in babies of around 3–5 months of age.

Short feeds do count as feeds. Babies become very efficient on the breast as they get bigger, and often only feed for a short amount of time – especially if there is a lot going on. Older babies may prefer a faster flow of milk, so sometimes they might want to go back on the breast a bit later, swap breasts with their twin, or need the parent to use breast compressions to help keep them interested for longer. Sometimes they might just want a two-minute feed from one breast and that is fine. They can actually transfer quite a large volume of milk in a short amount of time when they are older. They often prefer longer feeds at night when there is less going on, or when they are sleepy (e.g. just waking from a nap) in the daytime.

Unfortunately, some babies refuse completely. After three months breastfeeding becomes less of a reflex action and more of a choice for the baby. If a baby is overstimulated or overtired they often refuse to feed. Feeding to sleep sometimes stops working temporarily. These babies often feed fine at night and 'reverse cycle' so they take the majority of their milk intake during the night.

Nursing strikes are fairly common in the later stages of breast-feeding and are often caused by teething, illness, or another exterior factor. They are often mistaken for baby self-weaning but, if there is a sudden stop like this, especially if it is causing distress, it is more likely to be temporary and baby will begin to feed again with some coaxing.

Things parents can try if they experiencing this:

- Offer the breast when baby is sleepy and super chilled out. Just as baby is beginning to stir from a nap, before they're properly awake, often works well as it more resembles a night feed. Sometimes feeding lying down on the bed, or dimming the lights, can help.

- Do some skin to skin.

- Share a bath with baby. The warmth and skin to skin contact encourages them to feed.

- Offer a finger to suck, or a dummy if baby has one, then replace finger/dummy with the breast.

- Movement often encourages baby to latch. Parent can stand up and rock or sway and try to latch, or sit on the edge of the sofa or bed or on a birthing ball and bounce and try to latch. They can try feeding in the sling.

- Try to limit bottle use if at all possible. If baby really is not feeding for long periods, then giving some milk in another way would be appropriate, perhaps by spoon, cup, or paced bottle. Parents will need to pump to maintain milk production in this scenario.

- Be in an environment where other babies are breastfeeding. Babies love to copy.

The good news is that these babies tend to come back to breastfeeding after a few days or up to a week or two, so it should not be the end of their breastfeeding relationship. Occasionally babies do not restart breastfeeding and in this situation some parents will choose to continue to pump for their babies.

Breastfeeding babies with underlying health conditions

There are many underlying health conditions which may affect breastfeeding, from things that are fairly easy to fix such as tongue tie, to more serious complications. Here are some personal stories.

PERSONAL STORIES
Vikki with Joseph and Oliver

Finding out I was pregnant at 43 was a shock (contraception failure), finding out it was twins was a shock, and as these things come in threes we then found out one or both babies would have Down's syndrome (DS).

I felt I was a confident breastfeeder – I already had an 11 and 6-year-old, both of whom I exclusively breastfed until they were at least 12 months. Feeding twins would obviously be twice the work but I was adamant that is what I was going to do. We were researching how Down's syndrome was going to (possibly) affect our lives and too many times I read that babies with DS may not be able to breastfeed due to their low muscle tone, they may tire more easily due to heart conditions (50% of babies with DS have a heart issue), and a whole other list of reasons why it might not happen.

Joe and Olly were born at 37 weeks by planned C-section into a theatre full of people – twins require double staff anyway but because of the DS we had the paediatric team and cardiologists there too. There were approximately 20 people in the theatre and surrounding rooms! It was immediately apparent that Joe had Down's syndrome and Olly likely not (we still had to have the genetic tests done but it looked like we had a mismatched pair). To our delight Joe had no immediate health issues and came straight back to the ward with his twin and me.

Olly took to breastfeeding instantly – he was there and ready to go! Joe tried, he really tried, but his tongue was permanently pushed onto the roof of his mouth. We persisted – he wanted to breastfeed and I was determined to give him the best opportunity to do so. The benefits of breastfeeding a child with DS were documented and so important to me. Latching this tiny baby (4lb 6oz) on took forever – the timing to get a nipple in his tiny mouth at just the right time as his tongue moved down took some doing, then he would quite often slip off and he did fall asleep every time. We had a breastfeeding support nurse and she tried all the tricks, we undressed him, we blew on him, we tickled tiny feet to try and keep him awake, and used all the positions we could to try and make it work.

After two days on the ward being treated for jaundice Joe was diagnosed with polycythaemia (thick blood) and had to be rushed into NICU for immediate treatment – he had several bags of fluids by IV and as my milk was still not in he had to have formula feeds (the devastation was real but with no donor milk available and another baby still needing to feed I agreed). I made three-hourly visits to him as he progressed through NICU, HDU, and SCBU to put him on the breast. This was all day and all night. When I had no one to stay with Olly on the ward I used to walk him down through the corridors in his cot to see his brother! One night I was met by a very bemused security guard who had seen me on CCTV wandering the corridors in my nightgown at 3am, pushing a baby around and he rushed up to see what was going on!

Joe spent three days in the special care ward and, with my milk finally in and the assistance of two wonderful nurses to manhandle the nipple into his mouth, he finally had his first full feed with no top ups! From then on he was exclusively breastfed – for the first 8–10 weeks we still had issues with latching and slipping off but every feed was exercise for his muscles and improved things. Finally he became a breastfeeding pro – this boy could latch in the dark, from 30 paces out it seemed! Both boys ended up being successfully breastfed until three years eight months for Olly and four years for Joe! He still had a bedtime feed for a couple of months after starting school in September 2020.

Julia with Arthur and Violet

My twins were born at 37+1 by planned section. We knew that there was a problem with Arthur's heart and had been told that he would be taken quickly to the NICU. I was determined to try to feed, but also knew that it might not be possible for him. I managed to hand express over a hundred 1ml syringes of colostrum before they were born which I dropped off on my way to theatre. I wanted to do something for him and I felt that this was all I could do.

Once he was born I got to kiss his head before he disappeared. There were not the precious moments of skin to skin, that tiny person rooting for their first feed. I had that with Violet and it was all the more precious and poignant because Arthur was not there. There was nothing I could do for him and I felt so helpless. I didn't see him again for six hours and didn't get to hold him until he was two days old. I fed Violet who luckily proved to be a milk monster and was quickly encouraged to start using the hospital pump for Arthur. The staff soon asked if he could have donor milk and I readily agreed.

At seven days we moved to another hospital and Arthur was prepped for surgery. I had not yet been able to even put him to the breast, but my milk was in and I was keeping up with his needs as well as Violet's. I pumped every time I fed her, and I fed her a lot! Arthur had his first open heart surgery at nine days old, and spent nearly three weeks in intensive care because he didn't recover how they expected. During this time I filled their freezers. The doctors and dieticians insisted that some of his feeds (all tube) be high calo-rie formula but he still had some of my milk. He had been very poorly and was weak so needed any help he could get. At five weeks I was allowed to try and feed him directly. He wasn't really interested and just licked me. The next time I was allowed to offer (once a day) I tried with nipple shields and he did really well. I fed Violet at the same time and she triggered the let-down when his suck wasn't strong enough. I fed him once a day for the next couple of weeks.

After a week Arthur deteriorated and I persuaded the cardiol-ogist to let me feed him all day instead of using the high calorie formula. His saturation levels were better when I fed him and he was more stable. I was proved right, and the next months were filled with feeding plans and top ups through the tube. We still hadn't made it home. Violet and I were living in a room at the hospital and spending every waking moment on the ward with Arthur. We were not allowed to stay the night with him until they took his tube out at four months. They mistakenly thought he would take their high calorie formula from a bottle overnight, but he wouldn't and I wouldn't let them put the tube back.

After another surgery, another period of expressing for his feeds and struggling with supply, and another three months in hospital, we made it home. He was still having tube top ups. By this time they were nearly nine months old, and the tube didn't help him with eating solids so when he pulled it out we left it out.

That was two years ago, and we are still feeding with no signs of stopping. Breastfeeding a child through everything Arthur has been through was important for me as a mother. At times it was all I could do for him. I would sit next to him hoping and praying he would make the next day, with my plastic best friend pumping away and Violet my constant companion and shining light in my arms in my darkest moments. Feeding him meant that Violet and I could stay on the wards with him for the majority of his stays.

What to expect after the first few weeks

It is important to remember that all babies are individuals, even within a set of multiples who were born on the same day. Even if they are identical twins there can be quite a wide variation in their development. Babies are born with their own personality, partly genetic and partly influenced by the environment around them, both inside and outside the womb, and this can mean they have different ways of dealing with life. It's quite normal for one to need a little more support than the other. Many multiple birth parents feel torn in two or three directions and worry that perhaps one of their babies may be getting less attention because they are more settled. It's important to remember that some babies just do find life a bit easier, and they will soon tell you if they are not happy. Multiples do have to wait for things a bit more than most singletons, and this can be quite distressing for parents, but being near, singing, bouncing, talking to the babies while they are having to wait for their nappy change or whatever means they know the parent is there, and they know the parent is trying their best! There is no such thing as the perfect parent! Especially with more than one baby to care for, perfection does not exist. A good enough parent is just fine.

There are, however, certain patterns of development that are very common at certain times. As mentioned before, premature babies often reach these milestones somewhere between their actual age and their adjusted age, so the timings can be quite difficult to predict. Of course, even full term babies have a wide range of normal. So as long as the parents are following babies' lead as best they can, that is the most important thing.

Babies can be a bit fussy, feed a lot, wake more at night, and be more resistant to being put down than usual during these fussy periods. They often occur somewhere around three weeks, six weeks, three months, four months, six months, eight months etc. These fussy periods are often referred to as growth spurts, but are likely to be due to brain growth as well as body growth – developmental leaps. Parents often worry that they have not got enough milk during these periods and it is a common time to introduce formula. Reassuring them that if they can hang in there, clear the diary, and feed as much as possible then the fussy period usually passes quite quickly and milk production keeps up, is very important.

At around one month to six weeks, probably adjusted age for premature babies, we say milk production is fully established. What we mean by this is that research shows that between the age of one month and six months, a baby's 24-hour milk intake remains relatively constant. After six months, once solids are introduced, milk intake gradually reduces (Kent *et al.* 1999). Of course it may vary a little from day to day, but it does not continue to increase as some people think. This can be very encouraging to those who have managed to make a full milk production for their babies in the first few weeks.

However, there does not seem to be a cut-off point for increasing production at six weeks. It is often wrongly suggested that if a parent has not managed to make a full milk supply by around this age then it will not be possible. This is not the case. It is definitely possible to continue to increase supply, and especially if the babies are beginning to feed more effectively, any early feeding or latching issues have been resolved, and pumping and topping up can be reduced. With good support many parents find their production can catch up with their babies' intake. This is illustrated by the statistics gathered from the Breastfeeding Twins and Triplets UK Facebook group each year. Exclusive breastfeeding rates from those parents surveyed in 2015–19, rose from 35.5% at birth through to 46% at six weeks and on to 58% at 5–6 months (before solids were introduced). And combination feeding using formula fell from 40% at birth to 32% at six weeks and on to 20% at 5–6 months.

Babies gradually become more alert and as the weeks go past they spend more time awake. From around two months they often start to have wakeful periods after a feed, and then have more consolidated naps in between. These naps are often short, just one sleep cycle of around 40 mins in total, and if baby has fed to sleep half of this sleep cycle may be during the feed. Babies start to play a bit more at this age, and this is a lovely time for parents as they start to get rewarded with smiles and sounds. They also begin to develop their circadian rhythm at this age, starting to learn the difference between night and day, and can often sleep a little better with some longer stretches. Most babies will continue to wake for feeds but will be easier to settle afterwards. Some may even sleep through.

Somewhere between three and five months of age there is a really big period of fast development. Babies are learning so many new things and this can make them very distractible and unsettled. They often have short feeds and come on and off the breast frequently, and short naps are the norm. Sometimes they begin to refuse feeds, especially if they are tired. Feeding to sleep can become more challenging. But, once settled, if the parents try again they will often latch. Rocking, swaying, or bouncing while latching babies can help to get them to feed. Or this can be a good time to prioritise breast-feeding as babies begin to stir from a nap, before they are properly awake. Sleepy feeds are often more successful. Babies of this age are also changing their sleep patterns and can have more difficulty transitioning between the different sleep states. This can mean more night waking, or babies being more difficult to settle in the night.

Rhythms and routines

As you can see, babies change all the time. Parents often ask when it will be a good time to put their babies into a routine. There is a myth that a strict schedule is the only way to cope with more than one baby. It's true that there are babies who like to do a similar thing each day and fit into the routines that the books say they should, but there are many babies who really do not. Trying to make a baby sleep when it does not want to sleep, or trying to make them stretch out their feeds to three- or even four-hourly, just does not work at all. Parents can find this very stressful and feel that they are failing as a parent because their babies are not doing what the book tells them they should be doing. One study found that the use of baby books promoting strict routines for infant sleep, feeding, and general care was associated with increased depressive symptoms and stress, alongside lower self-efficacy. The majority of parents in this study did not find these baby books useful (Harries & Brown 2019). For some parents a routine may work but, for the majority, responsive parenting is likely to be preferable.

A simple bedtime routine can be helpful. In the early days this should be nothing complicated, and definitely should not be at a set time. Something as simple as dimming the lights, nappy change, dress in a clean babygrow, and feed to sleep is often sufficient. Other elements like a song, story, bath, or massage can be added in as the baby develops. A similar pattern of behaviour each bedtime signals to the baby that it is the end of the day and it is time for sleep, and can reinforce their circadian rhythm. In the first few months babies usually have a late bedtime and go to bed with their parents. Some may begin to need an earlier bedtime after a few months but until six months old they should be in the same room as an adult for all sleeps, for protection against SIDS.

Babies do get into general patterns of behaviour that can last a couple of weeks. Some will nap at a similar time each day for a while, until their sleep needs change. Twins and triplets can be encouraged to be in sync with their naps by feeding them at the same time, waking one when the other asks to feed. This often works well for the first part of the day but, as the afternoon leads into evening and the babies become more unsettled and fussy, it becomes more challenging to keep them in sync. Remember, babies' needs change all the time and so a pattern may work for a bit but perhaps the following week it will no longer. Babies' needs may have changed.

Ideally, a compromise of trying to be as responsive as possible alongside encouraging the babies to do some things at the same time is usually the best option. Being totally baby-led as a multiple birth parent can mean you literally have no time to even shower, but strict routines are also often not suitable – somewhere in between works well.

Top Tips for Parents

It is important to continue to feed and parent responsively.

Babies often continue to want to feed frequently but they do tend to get more efficient and feeds often become shorter.

You may notice patterns of feeding, naps, and behaviour which may last a few days or weeks.

Babies are changing and developing in all the time. The only certainty with babies is that they will be different next month from how they are now.

Babies will have periods of fussy behaviour where they ask to feed a lot and are unsettled in between. This is developmental and nothing that you are doing wrong. Try to roll with it and it will pass. Have a baby moon in front of the TV.

Night waking is normal. Babies continue to need feeding regularly overnight. There will be periods where the babies sleep for longer stretches and there will be times where they are waking more frequently. These are generally developmental. Try to follow their needs and maximise your own sleep whenever you can. Ask for support from others if you are struggling.

Try to live in the moment, cope with whatever they are doing now. Try not to worry about what will happen in the future as they will be totally different babies later on doing totally different things.

If something is working for you, keep doing it. It is nobody else's business how you care for your babies. If something is not working try something different. If that makes life easier keep doing it; if it makes it more difficult, try something else, or go back to what you were doing in the first place.

A baby's 24-hour milk intake stays roughly constant from around one month to six months. Their feeding patterns will change with time but the volume stays about the same.

If formula is introduced try to keep it to roughly the same time each day and breastfeed responsively the rest of the time.

As babies get older they often get more distracted when they feed. Night feeds are often better. Sleepy daytime feeds after a nap can help.

If something does not seem right, or if you are worried, ask for support. Many areas have breastfeeding support groups where you can drop in and have a chat. Breastfeeding helplines are also great. For more in depth support Breastfeeding Counsellors and IBCLCs can help.

Chapter 9

Breastfeeding Older Babies and Toddlers

Once established, many families find that continuing to breastfeed is an incredibly easy and fulfilling way of meeting their children's needs. Breastfeeding is the answer to many problems an older baby or toddler may encounter. It is a great way to settle them to sleep for naps or at night, helps comfort with bumps, scrapes, and illness, keeps them protected from illness when starting childcare, and helps regulate all those big emotions. Breastfeeding is a very effective parenting tool and stopping, especially if establishing breastfeeding was difficult in the early days, often just seems insane.

The World Health Organization recommends that families worldwide exclusively breastfeed infants for the child's first six months to enjoy optimal growth, development, and health. Thereafter they should be given nutritious complementary foods and continue breastfeeding up to the age of two years or beyond (World Health Organization 2011). Breast milk continues to be a nutritious element of a toddler's diet and the health benefits for both child and parent continue until whatever age breastfeeding ceases.

Introducing solid foods

Since 2001 the World Health Organization has recommended that babies can begin to be offered complementary solid foods alongside their milk feeds from around the age of six months (World Health Organization 2021). This is primarily based on health evidence but also takes into account a baby's physical development when several signs of readiness can be noted.

For premature babies the signs of readiness may occur a little later than six months actual age. BLISS suggests babies often show these signs that they are ready for solid foods somewhere between five and six months corrected age, and it is recommended to wait until you see a few of these signs before starting solids (BLISS 2021). In my experience most premature babies reach these milestones before six months adjusted age and starting somewhere between six months actual age and six months adjusted age, when babies are showing the following signs of readiness, makes for a more straightforward experience.

Signs of readiness are generally agreed upon as:

- Sitting with minimal support and being able to hold their head steady.

- Being able to reach, grab and bring food to their mouths.

- Their tongue thrust reflex, the protective reflex that pushes unwanted items out of baby's mouth, should have gone and baby should be able to bite some soft food, chew, and swallow.

- They should have an interest in food but this alone is not enough to start solids, they need to have the physical development in order to eat safely.

Amy Brown states in her book *Why Starting Solids Matters*:

In other words, the baby goes through a series of developmental stages, both in terms of internal digestive ability and external physical feeding skills. In most babies, by around six months these combine to enable babies to self-feed and digest food. Magic! (Brown 2017, p.48)

A baby beginning to wake more at night or wanting to feed more frequently is not a sign that they need to start solids, though it is commonly suggested that it may be. In fact it is a sign that they want to breastfeed more. Waiting for the signs of readiness for solids is important, whether the parents introduce puree, finger food, or a mixture.

In the first few months babies may only eat tiny amounts. It is all about play and exploration and getting messy. A baby's natural iron stores do start to decrease at around six months but they do not disappear overnight. However, when starting solids it can be a good plan to prioritise some of the more iron-rich foods such as eggs, meat, fish, and pulses. A wide variety of foods can be offered from six months of age, and babies can join in with family meals. Only if there is a history of food allergies, or if baby is already allergic to some foods through the parent's milk, should more caution be used. In this scenario introducing common allergens one at a time and watching for a reaction can be a good idea. However, the majority of babies can eat almost anything.

Foods to avoid:

- too much salt – not good for baby's kidneys

- added sugar – babies do not need it

- honey – risk of botulism

- mouldy or unpasteurised cheese – risk of listeria

- whole nuts – choking hazard

- whole grapes/cherry tomatoes etc. – choking hazard; should be cut into quarters lengthways

- raw meat and fish – should always be thoroughly cooked

- shark, swordfish, and merlin – high in mercury

- runny egg should be avoided (if not lion stamped in the UK or equivalent).

Some babies will take to food very quickly and eat larger portions. For these babies it is important to continue to prioritise milk feeds, as milk still forms the main part of their nutrition right up until the end of the first year. Other babies will only have small amounts for many months, and this is also within the normal range. We do not need to suggest the parents restrict milk feeds to encourage more solids as milk is far more nutrient dense than most foods. It is fine for them to take their time. The average baby seems to start to eat a bit more at around 9-10 months of age and this is the time they sometimes begin to cut back on their milk feeds a little.

Top Tips for Parents

Wait until babies have reached all the signs of readiness needed to start solids. It will be a much easier journey if the babies are developmentally ready to eat.

Signs of readiness include sitting fairly independently, being able to reach, grab, and bring food to their mouths, tongue thrust reflex reduced so babies can bite chew and swallow foods.

This is generally around six months for full term babies, but it does not matter if it is a little later.

For premature babies the signs of readiness normally occur between six months actual age and six months adjusted age.

Babies waking up more, breastfeeding more, watching you eat, or having slow weight gain are not reasons for starting solids early.

Share family foods. This is so much easier as it means babies get used to family foods and you only have to cook once.

Eat as a family wherever possible. Babies like to copy modelled behaviour, and eating is a social occasion in most societies.

Leave out the salt until after you have dished up the babies' portions.

Cut veg and meat into chip shapes so they are easy to hold. Babies will bite off the end.

If you prefer you can puree or mash the food. For sloppy foods such as soup or yoghurt babies can be given a preloaded spoon and encouraged to join in, so they can learn to feed themselves. They can also dip toast or bread sticks.

If you prefer to eat later with your partner then cook some extra so baby can have it the next day. It's good for babies' development if you sit down with them and join in with their mealtimes, even if you just have a drink.

From six months babies can eat pretty much anything except honey, runny egg (although if lion stamped it is safe), unpasteurised cheese, and whole nuts. Be adventurous!

Keep salt and sugar to a minimum.

Herbs and spices are fine. Babies often really enjoy strong flavours and a bit of spice.

Cut grapes, cherry tomatoes, and similar sized foods lengthways into quarters.

Expect some throwing – part of babies exploring foods is seeing what happens when it goes anywhere but in their mouths.

Most of all, have fun and embrace the mess! It is wonderful watching your babies explore and feed themselves.

Returning to work

It is important to know that returning to work does not mean you have to stop breastfeeding. It is totally possible to return to work and continue to breastfeed when you are together. How parents approach this depends very much on how old the babies will be when the parent returns to work.

Many parents are worried about how the caregiver will settle their babies to sleep without the magic of breastfeeding. Some babies will settle with a bottle, some with a cuddle, some with movement. Professional caregivers are normally very experienced with this scenario, and babies will tolerate settling in other ways far more when the breasts are not available. Babies who will only feed to sleep when with their parent are often fine to settle in another way in a childcare environment. If there are other children in the setting, such as at a nursery or busy childminder, then group mentality often kicks in. If the other babies are already sleeping, it is quite likely a newly-arrived baby will join them. Sometimes they may need some gentle interventions to begin with, while they get used to the new environment, but they generally settle with a bit of time. If family members are looking after them then it is important to empower them to find their own way of doing things. Babies can be cuddled for naps, patted or stroked, or taken out in the buggy or sling.

Under six months

If breastfeeding parents are returning to work before the babies are six months old then milk feeds are still their sole source of nutrition, and so pumping is likely to be a consideration. As soon as the parent is coming up to the time they plan to return to work they will need to contact their place of work to discuss the situation. Depending on the laws of the country, pumping breaks may be something that is protected or may not. Discussing up front what parents wish to do is important. Parents will need to make their own informed choice about whether they want to keep their babies exclusively breast milk fed, or whether they will introduce some formula. If they decide to keep their babies on breast milk then some considerations are needed.

Parents may want to pump a small stash of expressed milk so that they have some ready for the first day and some spare to give them a cushion in case pumping is difficult. Pumping is often not as efficient as directly breastfeeding, and some parents may find it difficult to express as much milk as the babies take directly. Preparing in advance can help give the parents confidence that their babies will have enough breast milk for the working week. Storing a little each day in the run up to the return to work will ensure they have some milk, while not being too time consuming or risking developing an oversupply.

Maximise breastfeeding when the parent and children are together. Making sure the babies feed directly as much as possible when with their parent will mean that milk supply is much easier to maintain. When babies are separated from their main caregiver in the daytime, they often start to wake a little more at night – this is known as 'reverse cycling'. Using this to maximise night feeds can help protect milk supply, so it is something to be encouraged (though waking more at night is hard for the newly returned-to-work parent). Co-sleeping and feeding lying down can make this more manageable. If the babies are able to be in a care setting near to the parent's work then they may be able to breastfeed the babies in breaks. Even one feed at lunchtime can make it easier to maintain milk supply. Ensure that the caregiver does not give a bottle feed just before the babies are due to be picked up by the parent, so that the babies can breastfeed straight away. Ensure caregivers know how to pace the bottle feeds to make sure babies do not take too much milk. This can mean that the parent does not need to express as much.

Breastfeeding parents are likely to need to pump their milk at roughly the times the babies would have fed if they were breastfeeding directly in order to maintain their milk supply. A hospital grade double pump can make this as efficient as possible, however sometimes it can be difficult to use these pumps in certain working environments. A more discreet pump that fits inside the parent's bra can be a good option. With these wearable pumps it is barely possible to tell that someone is pumping. They are not as efficient as a hospital grade pump, but it is better to pump using one of these pumps than not pump! On days that the parent is not working, maximising breastfeeding opportunities can boost supply for the following week. They could also try to pump once or twice a day to put get a bit of a head start for the next working days.

Between six and nine months

Babies should be starting to receive some solid food at this stage, which can take the pressure off the amount of expressed milk a parent will need to provide. However, milk continues to be the main source of nutrition, and the volumes of food ingested to begin with can be quite minimal. Babies should also be introduced to some water from a cup alongside their solid foods. All the same considerations need to be taken into account as for returning to work before six months: maximising breastfeeding when together, reverse cycling, making sure babies have not just had a feed before pick up, ensuring paced bottle feeding etc.

Babies of this age are often more resistant to taking a bottle and actually do not need to use one. Other ways of giving expressed milk can be explored. Often breastfed babies do better with an open cup; sometimes they are ok with a free-flowing sippy cup. Sometimes they will take some milk from a spoon. It's not unusual for babies to take a minimal amount of milk from another source, just enough to keep them going through the day, and then make up for it when reunited with the parent, cluster feeding after pick up and feeding frequently through the night – reverse cycling again. This can make it easier on the parent as they will not have to express as much milk but it can also be quite intense and exhausting!

Nine months and older

Solid foods will be much more established at this age and this can mean the return to work is far more straightforward. Babies of this age are often fine with just food and water during the day and then breastfeeding as normal when reunited, for any night feeds and first thing in the morning. On days together they can feed more in the day and the parent's supply will flex to accommodate this. Parents can choose to express at work if the babies enjoy a bottle or cup of milk, but it is not essential, and from a nutritional point of view they are likely to take all the milk they need at the times when they are together with the parent. Milk production can take a little time to adjust to the new pattern, so parents may feel a bit full by the end of the day and prefer to express for comfort to begin with. This is especially important if they have been prone to blocked ducts and mastitis in the past. Often the big cluster feeding session when reunited will sort out any engorgement. Wearing a dark top and breast pads can be a good plan, as parents may begin to leak again when they have not done so for a while. Breasts really do seem to know which day of the week it is – once the new routine has been established for a few weeks the breasts will adjust to the different feeding patterns and parents find they no longer feel engorged but there continues to be plenty of milk on their days together. They are very clever! Milk supply continues to work on a demand and supply basis, even across a week.

Working night shifts

Parents who have to work night shifts are often very worried about how their partner or other caregiver will cope without being able to feed the babies back to sleep. Giving expressed milk may help settle the babies, but often it is cuddles that replace breastfeeding in this scenario – the cuddles trigger the same sleepy oxytocin release as breastfeeding does, albeit to a lower amount. Sometimes partners may find that bed-sharing with the babies will help them to settle more easily.

Deciding to add formula or cow's milk

Some parents may make the decision to use formula on their return to work. However, this does not mean that they need to stop breastfeeding completely. They can continue to breastfeed when together, on pick up, in the night, and before leaving for work. Parents may decide to keep the same pattern of formula feeding on the days when they are not at work or they may continue to breastfeed fully on those days. Again, after a few weeks breasts will begin to know which days they need to produce more milk. Children over one year can have full fat cow's milk (or an appropriate non-dairy alternative) as a drink when the parent is at work, or have water to drink and get the necessary nutrition from the solid foods in their diet.

PERSONAL STORIES
Helen with Robyn and Marley

I returned to work when the girls had just turned six months. I shared my maternity leave with my wife, who took over the baton from me for the remaining four months until the summer holidays (both teachers). Going into the transition, I felt a plethora of emotions: gratitude that it was my wife as primary caregiver and not nursery just yet, guilt they wouldn't be ok (they were), fear I wouldn't be ok (I was) and a lot of anxiety about how feeding would go, due to the ingrained feeling of worry that they wouldn't put on weight still lingering from the first few weeks and months. In a whirlwind of unease and uncertainty, one thing was clear; I knew I wanted to continue breastfeeding and, after a challenging start, I was determined to get to the stage where feeding felt easy and lovely!

At the beginning I was expressing three times a day, trying to yield 600–750ml a day; enough for my wife to give three bottles each twin per day. I sent myself a bit stir crazy with this and encountered blebs, blocked ducts, and supply issues, spiralling me back to the painful issues I had at the beginning of my feeding journey. With some excellent support from friends, family, Breastfeeding Twins and Triplets UK and my post-natal doula-turned-friend, I managed to keep going and get through that bit. When the girls turned nine months, I saw an infant feeding specialist who threw out a little gem, suggesting I express for comfort and for my wife to offer some milk in the bottom of an open cup, and we ditch the bottles. We did, and after that we didn't look back! My supply settled, the girls took the milk from me that they wanted before and after school and my boobs adjusted accordingly...like magic!

I was soon then able to ditch the expressing (colleagues will miss the familiar sound from telephone and video meetings I'm sure!) and now the girls just take what they need when we're together and...feeding is easy and lovely!

Top Tips for Parents

If babies are still exclusively breastfed or have only just started solids they will need some milk during the day. You can choose to express your milk at work, or to introduce some formula.

If babies are well established on solids they may be fine with no milk during the day or a minimal amount.

Prioritise direct breastfeeding as much as possible. If you are already combination feeding prioritise breastfeeding when you are together.

Expect some reverse cycling behaviour. Night waking often increases with big changes of routine. Plus they miss you.

Breastfeeding is about connection and security as well as nutrition, so babies may increase their feeds when you are together until they get used to the new routine.

You only need a stash for the first day and possibly a bit extra as security. You can pump at work and give your baby that milk the next day.

If babies need milk feeds during the day, you can arrange to be able to pump at work. Make sure you have somewhere private to pump and somewhere to store the milk.

Babies will often take a minimal amount of milk, just enough to keep themselves going.

If babies are not having milk during the day you may find you need to hand express or pump a little for comfort to begin with, but your breasts should adjust quite quickly to the new routine.

Ensure you wear a dark colour; take a change of top in case you leak; a jacket, cardigan, or scarf can cover milk stains; using breast pads may be sensible. If you feel a let-down sensation and you cannot express, put pressure on the breast and press into the chest wall for a few seconds and it should prevent leaking.

If you decide to use formula you can continue to breastfeed when you are with your babies. Your breasts will adjust to the new requirements quite easily.

Breastfeeding and biting

This is a concern for many breastfeeding parents. What happens when my baby gets teeth?

Generally it's not a problem. If a baby is actively feeding then their tongue should cover the lower teeth, making it impossible for them to bite. Top teeth can rub a little, but they usually come through later than the bottom ones. Trying a more exaggerated latch, so pointing the nipple towards the nose and encouraging baby to tilt their head, tucking their bum and shoulders in tight to your body should take pressure off the top teeth and make it more comfortable.

Unfortunately, sometimes babies do clamp down, especially when they're teething, and if they do it is really painful! Ideally it is a good plan to prevent babies from doing it in the first place if at all possible. Many babies clamp down at the end of the feed when the flow has slowed and they get a bit bored, so if the parent looks for signs of baby becoming distracted they can take them off the breast before they clamp down. If the baby needs more milk they can go back on with a deep latch. Some breast compressions may encourage them to feed actively again. If they bite again perhaps give them a teething toy instead.

Babies may clamp down at the start of the feed – sometimes because they do not actually want a feed or sometimes while they are waiting for the let-down reflex. If the latter, breast compressions can increase the flow of the milk to keep them interested.

If the baby does clamp down, the parent could try inserting a finger to break the seal, but they do risk the baby biting their finger too. Another option to get them to let go of the breast is to bring them closer in to the breast, gently blocking their nose so they have to open their mouth to breathe. If the parent tries to just pull them off, then they risk dragging baby's teeth down the breast. If baby breaks the skin then moist wound healing will help heal it quickly.

Babies do not understand that biting hurts. In fact sometimes they find it quite amusing if the parent yelps and makes a funny noise when they bite. This may mean they try it again to see if they can provoke the same funny noise again, like playing with a squeaky toy. Trying not to react, if at all possible, will help prevent this, although that is easier said than done of course!

If babies continue to bite, take them off every time they do it or look like they are going to do it. They will soon learn not to bite the breast that feeds them. Thankfully it is usually a short phase!

Top Tips for Parents

Watch for signs baby is going to bite.

Take baby off before it happens.

Try offering the other breast, the faster flow may keep them interested.

If baby does not want a feed, try again a bit later.

If baby does clamp down, try inserting a finger, although you risk them biting your finger too, or try bringing them in closer to the breast so they have to open their mouth and let go to breathe.

Try not to yelp as it can become a game (easier said than done!).

If baby is teething, offer pain relief about half an hour before a feed. Offer something cold to chew on as an alternative if they bite.

Moist wound healing will help any break in the skin heal quickly.

It is usually a short phase!

Nursing manners

Some babies and toddlers try lots of different behaviours when they are feeding. Things like pinching, twiddling the other nipple, or kneading the breast to increase the flow, grabbing hair, putting their hands in the parent's mouth, coming on and off, trying to stand up while they feed and all sorts of other acrobatics. And for twins who are tandem feeding there is the added distraction of their sibling within arm's reach. They can end up pulling their sibling's hair, poking them in the eye, or even taking the breast out of their sibling's mouth. Sometimes they like to swap sides with their sibling over and over again. Some of these behaviours are cute. Some hurt. Some are just downright annoying!

It is important to remember that although these behaviours are normal, if the parent is finding something intolerable, nursing is a two-, or three-, or four-way relationship. The parent does have a say in what is ok. They really do not have to put up with it.

Start early. If the toddlers begin to do something that the parent does not like, start to work on it immediately. Many behaviours are just temporary while they learn and explore, but if it is something the parent cannot stand, it is important to nip it in the bud in case it becomes ingrained.

Distraction is by far the most effective tool. If it is a behaviour involving the child's hand, giving them something else to hold or play with can keep them busy during a feed. This could be a toy, a scarf, or a necklace perhaps. Or you can move their hand away onto a less sensitive part of the body or away from their siblings. Using language such as 'gentle hands' and modelling a gentle touch can help them understand that pinching or scratching or poking the parent or sibling is not acceptable.

Offer an alternative to feeding if the behaviour does not stop. Perhaps the parent could take them off the breast and offer a toy or a teether to chew, or a snack or drink instead. They may want to swap sides. If they are feeding on their own, they will get a faster flow from the other breast, but sometimes when tandem feeding a change of side and position can also do the trick.

Use some gentle discipline. If the unwanted behaviours continue, take them off the breast and explain simply that it hurts or the parent does not like it. If they want to continue to feed they need to stop. Even quite young toddlers have some understanding of basic language, although they may not like it!

Boundaries are important. Obviously if a child is doing something that hurts the parent they need to understand that this cannot continue. Explain gently that this hurts and they cannot do it. Having boundaries also starts to introduce the concept of body autonomy. The breast does belong to the parent after all, not the child. Of course we will feed our babies willingly whenever they ask, but as they get older it is a good way to introduce the concept that they do not have complete control over the parent's body, they need consent. Once this concept is introduced, the child can also use this themselves with their own bodies. Multiple birth toddlers have to understand this concept earlier than most as they have a sibling or siblings of the same age who may display many behaviours towards them that they do not like, or may not like some of the behaviours displayed by the child. Again modelling gentle touch, asking before they touch or take things, and explaining how the other may feel are all concepts multiple birth parents have to explain 24 hours a day, not just at nursery or playgroup. It is exhausting but, with all this extra practice, multiple birth toddlers often become skilled at sharing and being empathic earlier than their singleton contemporaries.

Use a code word or sign for them to ask to feed. Some parents find the way their child asks to nurse difficult. They may shout 'Boobie!' at the top of their voices across the room, or they may start to help themselves by grabbing clothing, undoing a bra strap, putting their hands down the parent's top. This can be quite embarrassing in certain situations. Developing a sign or code word that is more acceptable can make the situation easier to deal with, especially when in public.

Some toddlers really are quite obsessed with breastfeeding and nurse very frequently throughout the day, and this can be quite difficult to deal with. During the 2021 lockdown many parents of nursing toddlers reported that their child had increased feeds because they were in the house all day, working from home with few distractions. Distraction is by far the best way to curb incessant toddler feeding. Going out to play, going to toddler groups, meeting with friends with children, keeping them busy with interesting activities are all effective. Offer drinks and snacks as an alternative to breastfeeding, they may be genuinely hungry or thirsty. Going out at nap time and having motion naps in the pushchair or car can prevent the need to feed to sleep.

Sleep into the toddler years

It is biologically normal for babies and toddlers to wake in the night for the first year or two, or even three. Many children do not reliably sleep through without any parental intervention until pre-school or school age. One study found that although there was a decrease in night waking after six months, 6–18-month-old infants continued to wake one to three times a night (Hysing *et al.* 2014). Teething can cause issues until all their molars have broken through, and illness often throws a spanner in the works. Development continues to have an effect, as do big changes in their lives such as the parents returning to work, starting nursery, or the arrival of a sibling.

Continuing to be as responsive as possible is ideal, as the child has a genuine need to be helped to fall back to sleep. Things to try to improve night time sleep include getting lots of exercise during the day, having some time each day where the parent gives the children their full attention, making sure naps are optimised, and a simple bedtime routine at a time that is suitable for the child. Very few children are genuinely sleep deprived, and the amount of total sleep a child needs varies widely from one child to the next. It can be difficult to compare, even from one multiple to the next. As they become older and more able to understand, parents can begin to explain their expectations and gradually be able to encourage them to become independent. Children often need sleep associations to settle – to be honest, adults often do too!

Night weaning multiples

Babies wake in the night. We know that. Babies like to feed a lot in the night. That's a given. But sometimes it all becomes too much. Sometimes it's exhaustion, sometimes it's nursing aversion, sometimes work commitments and sometimes it's just that mum has had enough. Night weaning is generally not recommended in the first year as the main source of nutrients continues to be milk during this time. It can be easier to night wean after 18 months as the babies will have a bit more understanding.

Breastfeeding is by far the easiest and fastest way to settle a baby back to sleep when they wake, but there may be a point where the parent needs to stop. This should be for them to decide and nobody else. They will know if they are ready to night wean. It is important to understand that night weaning will not necessarily make the babies sleep any better – they may still wake, and then the parents will have lost the easiest way to settle them back to sleep.

Breastfeeding at night is not so much about nutrition for toddlers, although human milk is of course still full of the same nutrients and immunological factors as in the early days. As babies grow into toddlers there is a big emotional context to these night feeds. Breastfeeding helps them feel safe, to deal with all the big emotions of being a toddler, to deal with the pain of teething, to reconnect after being separated due to work and childcare. There is a whole load going on. So it is important not to take away the other comforts that they are used to while you try to night wean – co-sleeping, bed-sharing, cuddles, a comforting toy. These can help the transition away from relying on the breast to settle back to sleep.

Should all the babies be night weaned together? Or should parents deal with them separately? This is a difficult one as it really depends on their own individual situation. Is one baby more settled than another? Or are they all equally wakeful? Will one baby be happy to settle for the partner or other helper? Are they bed-sharing? Do the babies have their own bedroom? Do they have separate rooms? There are all sorts of factors to take into account. If one baby is more settled, able to settle for a partner, or they are in separate rooms, then it may be easier to try night weaning separately. Otherwise it is often easier to do both together.

Parents can talk to their toddlers throughout the day about how breasts will be asleep tonight and how they can have some in the morning. Encourage them to consider an alternative. Let them choose which comforter they would like to use. Remind them again just before bedtime. Try to keep it positive and explain when they can feed again, rather than focusing on rejecting them and saying no, not now. There are several books aimed at toddlers that discuss night weaning and explain to the toddler that they will be able to nurse when the sun comes up. Reading these in the lead up to any changes can ease the transition.

It's a good idea to find other ways to help settle the toddlers at night. Lyndsey Hookway coined the phrase 'Habit Stacking' in her 2019 book *Holistic Sleep Coaching*. This is the concept of overlaying other sleep associations alongside the one the parents wish to stop, then gradually removing the association they no longer wish to use. There are many different things to try as alternative sleep associations and often a combination work well: cuddling, stroking, patting, singing, humming, use of a special toy or blanket, physical touch, holding hands, music, white noise, whatever works best for them. Some will work better than others, and everyone is different. Parents will find the best option for them, and they often have a few in place already. Twins and triplets also have a ready-made comforter: each other! One of the plus points of having more than one baby is that they do give comfort and security to each other. In the early days many parents co-bed their twins or triplets and find this can help with settling them to sleep. As they get older a lot of parents separate them, as they start to disturb each other, but sometimes when they are toddlers they may like to sleep together again, especially at times of transition.

One thing to try is to cuddle or stroke back to sleep while they are stirring before properly awake. Toddlers go through sleep cycles from deep, slow wave sleep to light rapid eye movement (REM) sleep regularly, and it is during the REM sleep that they often fully rouse and need help to resettle back into a deeper sleep again. Unfortunately a toddler's sleep cycle is shorter than an adult's, but if the parent can be aware the toddler is stirring and then cuddle or rest their hand on baby's body to help them settle before they are completely awake, they may find the toddler goes back into another deep sleep without fully waking and demanding to be fed. This is more effective if bed-sharing, as the adult will need to be in close proximity to be aware when they are about to wake. Sometimes turning baby away from the breast and cuddling tightly from behind works well, as they are less likely to want to latch if it is not right in their face.

Shortening feeds can be especially effective if you are experiencing nursing aversion. The negative feelings described as nursing aversion are often hormonally driven; ovulation and menstruation can be a trigger, and pregnancy is a major culprit. In order to continue being able to breastfeed, shortening the feeds can work well. Break the feed just before the toddler is about to drift off to sleep and encourage them to do that last bit on their own. You can always re-latch them if it doesn't work. Once the toddler is used to this you can gradually unlatch sooner and eventually they may settle to sleep from awake on their own. Some like to sing a song during this feed and when the song is finished, the feed is finished. Or count down to the end of the feed. If the parent is having a particularly bad day they can sing or count faster! Once the toddlers are good at settling to sleep without the breast they may be more able to move between their night time sleep cycles without feeding. They may drop off with just the song, or settle with just a few sucks.

Try with just one of the night feeds. The first wake-up of the night can be a good place to start – see if you can settle them in a different way. This is the most likely night feed to be able to drop more easily, because as the night progresses and morning approaches sleep often becomes lighter and toddlers are more difficult to settle back to sleep.

They often like to get up very early at this age. The most likely thing to help you stay in bed for a bit longer is to continue to breastfeed in the early mornings!

The other parent in a twin or triplet family is often much more hands on than in your average family, as there is much more to do! If toddlers are happy to settle with the other parent, and they must be truly happy, sometimes this can be a good technique to night wean. The partner can go in first and see if they can settle them – if it doesn't work then the breastfeeding parent can go in and breastfeed back to sleep. Some babies are more receptive to this than others. It may be that one of the babies is fine with the other parent and it is possible to night wean one of them easily, and then follow that by concentrating on the other. Sometimes the babies can be split up, with the non-breastfeeding parent taking one of the toddlers and sleeping with them, while the breastfeeding parent sleeps with the other. However, often only the breastfeeding parent will do, so if this is causing further distress it may be a good idea to stop. Remember, for a toddler breastfeeding is a way to connect with their most important person in the world, and keeping the connection is important.

Night weaning is often a very gradual process. Aiming for small goals and baby steps is more realistic than expecting big changes straight away. Parents should not be afraid to stop if weaning does not feel right. Teething, illness, and changes of circumstances can all increase night waking, and sometimes it may just be easier to go back to breastfeeding in the night again. Then once the unsettled period has passed parents can try again. Sometimes one or two night feeds are actually quite doable and continuing with these can actually make night times easier. Each journey is very personal between parent and children, and what will work for one family will not necessarily work for another.

Moving away from bed-sharing

Most families partially bed-share – either for part of the night, or on some nights and not others. Others find that bed-sharing is the only way to get some decent sleep and bed-share full time. It is biologically normal for babies and young children to share their parent's bed and there is no need to stop doing it if it is working for the family. Many babies will naturally start to settle more easily in their cot at some point, and the parents gradually stop bed-sharing as time goes on. However, some fully bed-sharing parents worry how they will ever get their older babies into their own room, and into their own cots. A cot is a Western invention and not actually necessary – there is another way which can be much easier, gentler, and less stressful for everyone: the floor bed.

The main difficulty of using a cot is having to lower the baby into it without waking them. Contrary to popular belief, many children under the age of two do not lie down and go to sleep happily on their own. Many still need a feed or a cuddle to do this. But getting them to go into the cot after feeding or cuddling to sleep can be difficult. As soon as you lower them down and let go, they're awake again – either almost straight away or at the end of the first sleep cycle. Having two or three babies to settle can take absolutely ages. A floor bed can remedy a lot of these problems: either just a mattress on the floor, or on a low slatted bed base, or in conjunction with a cot (or two) with the side taken off.

Here are some of the positives:

- Babies are settled to sleep in the bed they are expected to sleep in. Often a baby falls asleep in its parent's arms or bed as this is the easiest way to get them to sleep. Then, when the baby wakes up, they find themselves in their cot, sometimes in a different room. This can be very disorienting, as any adult who has woken somewhere different to where they fell asleep can testify!

- If the baby wakes in the night, the parent can settle them back to sleep in the baby's own bed easily with a feed or a cuddle. No need to move them out of their environment.

- The fact it is on the floor means it is safe if they roll out, or get up and wander in the night. And they will not try to climb out of the cot! The room should be childproofed by ensuring furniture is screwed to the walls for safety, nothing can be pulled on top of them, and there are no unsafe objects within reach. Some people find it helpful to put a baby gate on the bedroom door. A baby monitor can also be used.

- Parents can co-sleep part of the night in baby's bed if necessary, ensuring a good night's sleep for all. This also means that the other parent can remain in the parental bed. The co-sleeping parent can sneak back to their own bed if they are still awake once baby has settled.

- The floor bed is a very gentle way to encourage a baby to move into their own room or in with their sibling whenever the parents think this is the correct time for their family.

- Later on the parent can gradually retreat by lying next to the child, lying a bit further away, popping out for a minute, until eventually they are happy with a story, a kiss and a cuddle, and then sleep.

- For parents wanting a gentle way to transition a child to sleeping on their own space this can be an ideal solution.

Stopping breastfeeding toddlers

We probably all know that breastfeeding well into toddlerhood and beyond is recommended by the World Health Organization and that it is normal to do so (although this message still seems to be a bit slow to filter through to some!).

However, sometimes breastfeeding just isn't working for the parent. Maybe they have aversion, maybe they're feeling totally exhausted and touched out, maybe they're uncomfortable with still breastfeeding, maybe they just need to stop!

Breastfeeding is a two-way relationship and anyone who says a parent is breastfeeding their toddler for their own benefit has not breastfed a toddler. Especially if they are breastfeeding two or three toddlers! It is *intense*! They often seem to want to feed all day.

So the first step is try getting into a loose routine. A lot of parents find feeding first thing in the morning, mid-morning (before or after nap depending on whether they still feed to sleep), mid-afternoon (before or after nap), and bedtime works well, as well as maybe some night feeds of course. They may find just cutting back a bit like this and taking a bit more control makes continuing to feed more manageable and that they can keep going for a bit longer.

If the parent still wants to gradually wean then the easiest feed to drop is usually mid-morning, especially if they go out to baby groups or classes, as you can distract while out and the babies will tend to fall asleep on the way home in sling, car, or buggy. Have lunch ready for when they wake up. Once the babies have stopped having the mid-morning feed the parent could try stopping the mid-afternoon feed. Again, they could get ready with drink and snacks to combat the post-nap grumps if they happen.

Once they are down to morning and bedtime feeds, many people actually enjoy it again and hang on to those two feeds for a while. When they are ready to stop the early morning feed, the parent can just get up straight away and have breakfast. Being up and dressed before the babies will help with this transition.

For the bedtime feed the parent can gradually move away from feeding to sleep and then switch around the order of the bedtime routine. So instead of feeding to sleep or feeding as the last thing to settle, they could try feeding the babies first and then do teeth, pyjamas, story, and cuddle to sleep. This breaks the feed to sleep association and will make it much easier to then stop the feed completely.

Once a nursing parent has stopped feeding it is common for the drop in hormones to make them feel quite down, or even unwell, for a while. It takes the body a bit of time to adjust to the lower levels of oxytocin (which makes us feel good). Lots of cuddles will get the oxytocin flowing and help everyone adjust.

Breastfeeding to natural term

Feeding to natural term basically means continuing to breastfeed until the child is ready to stop themselves. It is commonly known as self-weaning. All children do eventually wean if they are left to their own devices. And the health benefits continue for everybody throughout the breastfeeding journey, no matter how long it is.

Breastfeeding into childhood is normal in many cultures around the world. Research shows that children will generally self-wean somewhere between two and a half and seven years old. Some children will self-wean under the age of two, but this is often because feeds have had to be limited due to work commitments for example, or due to a subsequent pregnancy reducing milk supply.

Self-weaning is generally a very slow, gentle decrease in feeding over a long period of time. It is not a sudden stop. If a baby refuses to feed suddenly that would be classed as a nursing strike, which is usually temporary and caused by an external factor such as illness or teething, however sometimes this becomes permanent and they do not start to feed again.

As the child grows older, feeding patterns often begin to become less frequent and more erratic. If they are ill, teething, hurt, or in a new, unfamiliar situation then they may ask to feed. If they are busy, happy, and distracted they are less likely to ask. As they begin to sleep more consistently, night feeds stop. Often bedtime and morning feeds continue for a long time. But maybe the child will stop feeding at bedtime at some point, or maybe start to sleep later in the morning so there's not time to feed before nursery or school. There are all sorts of scenarios. As the child starts to approach their natural weaning time, they don't always feed every day, or may even go up to a week or two without asking. They may just ask to feed on snuggly Sunday lie-ins, or if they are struggling to fall asleep.

When a child self-weans the parent often does not realise they have had a last feed. And then suddenly it has been several weeks since the child last asked. And then that is it. Or sometimes the child announces that they are no longer going to feed anymore!

PERSONAL STORIES
Sarah with Lowri and Caelan
Breastfeeding is my ultimate parenting tool.

I am in awe of the capabilities of my body to grow, birth, nourish, and comfort all of my children. I am child-led in all areas – I didn't potty train, they told me (at very different ages) when they were ready and were pretty immediately dry day and night. So deciding to follow their leads to their natural terms for breastfeeding, it feels right for me. Although I'm a little surprised that it has led to continuing to breastfeed five-year-olds in Year 1.

'Milky' provides untold depths of comfort and security for them. I'm reliably informed that 'Milky is my best friend', or told 'Mummy you sit there, I'll sit next to Milky'.

Breastfeeding verbal children is a revelation. Feeding twins who also have an impact on each other's feeding is such a different journey to the nearly four years I fed my older child.

I think it's possible one twin would have weaned earlier as a singleton. He is called in by the other twin. 'Come and get your milky!', 'You haven't had any yet. Mummy open your milky!' Twin led feeding and weaning has added complicating layers!

Top Tips for Parents

The only people who have a say in how long you feed your babies are you and your babies. Try to ignore any criticism from friends and family.

Human milk continues to have just as many health benefits to toddlers, pre-schoolers, and older children as it does in the early days. The health benefits for breastfeeding parents are often dose related, so the longer you feed the greater the protection.

Human milk contains antibodies to the particular viruses that are encountered by families. This can be useful when childcare bugs are going round.

Breastfeeding helps toddlers regulate big emotions, helps with pain relief for bumps and scrapes, helps overstimulated children calm down.

Night waking continues to be very common in the toddler years.

If feeding to sleep is still working for you then it is fine to continue.

If feeding to sleep is not working for you it may be time to try some gentle night weaning techniques. However, night weaning is not a guarantee that they will wake any less.

Adding some nursing manners can prevent unwanted behaviour and make it doable to continue to breastfeed. It is a two-, three-, or four-way relationship after all.

If aversion is creeping in, know that it is a common experience. If some feeds become unsustainable you can reduce or remove these and continue to breastfeed other less triggering feeds.

Distraction is the easiest way to wind down daytime breastfeeding.

Habit stacking other sleep cues and ways to settle back to sleep before removing feeding is a gentle way of night weaning that often works well.

Conclusion

I hope this book will give useful information and tools to health care professionals, breastfeeding supporters, and parents in order to help multiple birth families meet and even exceed their feeding goals. There are many barriers to establishing and maintaining breastfeeding when multiples are involved, but when good support is available these can mostly be overcome.

As parents of multiples it can be easy to feel discriminated against, as often more specialised support is necessary and this can be difficult to access, especially with a huge double buggy and several babies to deal with. Making support as easily accessible as possible will ensure that families who need it will be able to find it and use it.

Multiple birth families are not that common. But they are just as important as anyone else and deserve as much support to meet their feeding goals.

My final take-home thought – let's value every drop! However long breastfeeding continues, whether this is three days, three months, or three years; however much milk the babies receive, whether this is a few syringes of colostrum, combination feeding, or exclusive breastfeeding, feeding multiple babies is a massive achievement and should be applauded.

References

Acuña-Castroviejo, D., Escames, G., Venegas, C., Díaz-Casado, M. E. *et al.* (2014) Extrapineal melatonin: sources, regulation, and potential functions. *Cellular and Molecular Life Sciences*, 71(16), 2997–3025.

Akacem, L. D., Wright Jr, K. P. & LeBourgeois, M. K. (2016) Bedtime and evening light exposure influence circadian timing in preschool-age children: a field study. *Neurobiology of Sleep and Circadian Rhythms*, 1(2), 27–31.

Ayton, J., Hansen, E., Quinn, S. & Nelson, M. (2012) Factors associated with initiation and exclusive breastfeeding at hospital discharge: late preterm compared to 37 week gestation mother and infant cohort. *International Breastfeeding Journal*, 7(1).

Ball, H. L. (2006) Caring for twin infants: sleeping arrangements and their implications. *Evidence Based Midwifery*, 4(1), 10–16.

Ball, H. L. (2007) Together or apart? A behavioural and physiological investigation of sleeping arrangements for twin babies. *Midwifery*, 23(4), 404–12.

Bergman, N. J. (2013) Neonatal stomach volume and physiology suggest feeding at 1-h intervals. *Acta Paediatrica*, 102(8), 773–7.

Bergman, N. J., Linley, L. L. & Fawcus, S. R. (2004) Randomized controlled trial of skin-to-skin contact from birth versus conventional incubator for physiological stabilization in 1200- to 2199-gram newborns. *Acta Pediatrica*, 93(6), 779–85.

Biran, V., Decobert, F., Bednarek, N., Boizeau, P. *et al.* (2019) Melatonin levels in preterm and term infants and their mothers. *International Journal of Molecular Sciences*, 20(9), 2077.

BLISS (2021) How do I know if my baby is ready to wean? Available at www.bliss.org.uk/parents/about-your-baby/feeding/weaning-your-premature-baby/how-do-i-know-if-my-baby-is-ready-to-wean, accessed 11 May 2022.

Brisbane, J. M. & Giglia, R. C. (2013) Experiences of expressing and storing colostrum antenatally: a qualitative study of mothers in regional Western Australia. *Journal of Child Health Care*, 19(2), 206–15.

Brown, A. (2017) *Why Starting Solids Matters.* London: Pinter & Martin.

Brown, A. (2018) What do women lose if they are prevented from meeting their breastfeeding goals? *Clinical Lactation*, 9(4), 200–7.

Cavkll, B. (1981) Gastric emptying in infants fed human milk or infant formula. *Acta Paediatrica*, 70(5), 639–41.

Centers for Disease Control and Prevention (2020) How to keep your breast pump kit clean: the essentials. Available at www.cdc.gov/healthywater/hygiene/healthychildcare/infantfeeding/breastpump.html, accessed 11 May 2022.

Centers for Disease Control and Prevention (2021) Proper storage and preparation of breast milk. Available at www.cdc.gov/breastfeeding/recommendations/handling_breastmilk.htm, accessed 11 May 2022.

Clarke, P., Allen, E., Atuona, S. & Cawley, P. (2021) Delivery room cuddles for extremely preterm babies and parents: concept, practice, safety, parental feedback. *Acta Pediatrica*, 110, 1439–49.

De Carvalho, M., Robertson, S., Friedman, A. & Klaus, M. (1983) Effect of frequent breast-feeding on early milk production and infant weight gain. *Pediatrics*, 72(3), 307–11.

Fewtrell, M. S., Kennedy, K., Ahluwalia, J. S. *et al.* (2016) Predictors of expressed breast milk volume in mothers expressing milk for their preterm infant. *Archives of Disease in Childhood – Fetal and Neonatal Edition*, 101, 502–6.

Fieth, J. (2020) After weaning – what next? Available at www.laleche.org.uk/after-weaning-what-next, accessed 11 May 2022.

Flower, H. (2019) *Adventures in Tandem Nursing: Breastfeeding During Pregnancy and Beyond.* 2nd ed. Hilary Flower (self-published).

Forster, D. A., Moorhead, A. M., Jacobs, S. E., Davis, P. G. *et al.* (2017) Advising women with diabetes in pregnancy to express breastmilk in late pregnancy (Diabetes and Antenatal Milk Expressing [DAME]): a multicentre, unblinded, randomised controlled trial. *Lancet*, 389(10085), 2204–13.

Hackman, N. M., Alligood-Percoco, N., Martin, A., Zhu, J. & Kjerulff, K. H. (2016) Reduced breastfeeding rates in firstborn late preterm and early term infants. *Breastfeeding Medicine*, 11(3), 119–25.

Hallowell, S. & Spatz, D. (2012) The relationship of brain development and breastfeeding in the late-preterm infant. *Journal of Pediatric Nursing*, 27(2), 154–62.

Harries, V. & Brown, A. (2019) The association between use of infant parenting books that promote strict routines, and maternal depression, self-efficacy, and parenting confidence. *Early Child Development and Care*, 189(8), 1339–50.

Henderson, J., Hartmann, P., Newnham, J. & Simmer, K. (2008) Effect of preterm birth and antenatal corticosteroid treatment on lactogenesis II in women. *Pediatrics*, 121(1), 92–100.

Hill, P. D., Aldag, J. C., Chatterton, R. T. & Zinaman, M. (2005) Primary and secondary mediators' influence on milk output in lactating mothers of preterm and term infants. *Journal of Human Lactation*, 21(2), 138–50.

Hookway, L. (2019) *Holistic Sleep Coaching.* Amarillo, TX: Praeclarus Press.

Hookway, L. (2020) *Let's Talk About Your New Family's Sleep.* London: Pinter & Martin.

Hysing, M., Harvey, A. G., Torgersen, L., Ystrom, E., Reichborn-Kjennerud, T. & Sivertsen, B. (2014) Trajectories and predictors of nocturnal awakenings and sleep duration in infants. *Journal of Developmental & Behavioral Pediatrics*, 35(5), 309–16.

Jha, P., Morgan, T. A. & Kennedy, A. (2019) US evaluation of twin pregnancies: importance of chorionicity and amnionicity. *Radiographics*, 39(7).

Kato, I., Horike, K., Kawada, K., Htun, Y. *et al.* (2022) The trajectory of expressed colostrum volume in the first 48 hours postpartum: an observational study. *Breastfeeding Medicine*, 17(1), 52–8.

Kendall-Tackett, K., Cong, Z. & Hale, T. W. (2011) The effect of feeding method on sleep duration, maternal well-being, and postpartum depression. *Clinical Lactation*, 2(2), 22–6.

Kent, J. C., Mitoulas, L. R., Cregan, M. D., Ramsay, D. T., Doherty, D. A. & Hartmann, P. E. (2006) Volume and frequency of breastfeedings and fat content of breast milk throughout the day. *Paediatrics*, 117(3), 387–395.

Kent, J. C., Mitoulas, L., Cox, D. B., Owens, R. A. & Hartmann, P. E. (1999) Breast volume and milk production during extended lactation in women. *Experimental Physiology*, 84(2), 435–47.

Lawrence, R. A. & Lawrence, R. M. (2021) *Breastfeeding – A Guide for the Medical Profession*. 9th ed. New York: Elsevier.

López-Fernández, G., Barrios, M., Goberna-Tricas, J. & Gómez-Benito, J. (2017) Breastfeeding during pregnancy: a systematic review. *Women and Birth: Journal of the Australian College of Midwives*, 30(6), e292–e300.

Ludington-Hoe, S. M., Lewis, T. & Morgan, K. (2006) Breast and infant temperatures with twins during shared Kangaroo Care. *Journal of Obstetric, Gynecologic & Neonatal Nursing*, 35(2), 223–31.

Marasco, L. & West, D. (2019) *Making More Milk: The Breastfeeding Guide to Increasing Your Milk Production*. 2nd ed. New York: McGraw Hill.

MBRRACE (2021) *MBRACE-UK Perinatal Confidentiality Enquiry: Stillbirths and Neonatal Deaths in Twin Pregnancies*. Oxford: University of Oxford.

Meier, P. P., Brown, L. P., Hurst, N. M., Spatz, D. L. *et al.* (2000) Nipple shields for preterm infants: effect on milk transfer and duration of breastfeeding. *Journal of Human Lactation*, 16(2), 106–14.

Meier, P., Patel, A. L., Wright, K. & Engstrom, J. L. (2013) Management of breastfeeding during and after the maternity hospitalization for late preterm infants. *Clinical Perinatology*, 40(4), 689–705.

Mohrbacher, N. (2010) The 'magic number' and long-term milk production (parts I and II). Available at www.nancymohrbacher.com/articles/2010/8/13/the-magic-number-and-long-term-milk-production-part-1.html, accessed 11 May 2022.

Morton, J., Hall, J. Y., Wong, R. J., Thairu, L., Benitz, W. E. & Rhine, W. D. (2009) Combining hand techniques with electric pumping increases milk production in mothers of preterm infants. *Journal of Perinatology*, 29(11), 757–64.

Morton, J., Wong, R. J., Hall, J. Y., Pang, W. W. *et al.* (2012) Combining hand techniques with electric pumping increases the caloric content of milk in mothers of preterm infants. *Journal of Perinatology*, 32(10), 791–6.

Multiple Births Foundation (2019) Media enquiries/multiple birth statistics. Available at www.multiplebirths.org.uk/media.asp, accessed 11 May 2022.

NICE (2017) *Faltering Growth: Recognition and Management of Faltering Growth in Children NICE Guideline* [NG75]. London: National Institute for Health and Care Excellence.

NICE (2019) *Twin and Triplet Pregnancy NICE Guideline* [NG137]. London: National Institute for Health and Care Excellence.

Nyqvist, K. H. (2008) Breastfeeding Preterm Infants. In C. W. Genna (ed.) *Supporting Sucking Skills in Breastfeeding Infants.* Boston: Jones & Bartlett Learning.

Nyqvist, K. H., Sjödén, P. O. & Ewald, U. (1999) The development of preterm infants' breastfeeding behavior. *Early Human Development*, 55(3), 247–64.

Prime, D. K., Garbin, C. P., Hartmann, P. E. & Kent, J. C. (2012) Simultaneous breast expression in breastfeeding women is more efficacious than sequential breast expression. *Breastfeeding Medicine*, 7(6), 442–7.

Prime, D. K., Geddes, D. T., Hepworth, A. R., Trengove, N. J. & Hartmann, P. E. (2011) Comparison of the patterns of milk ejection during repeated breast expression sessions in women. *Breastfeeding Medicine*, 6(4), 183–90.

Ramsay, D. T., Mitoulas, L. R., Kent, J. C., Cregan, M. D. *et al.* (2006) Milk flow rates can be used to identify and investigate milk ejection in women expressing breast milk using an electric breast pump. *Breastfeeding Medicine*, 1, 14–23.

Saint, L., Maggiore, P. & Hartmann, P. E. (1986) Yield and nutrient content of milk in eight women breast-feeding twins and one woman breast-feeding triplets. *The British Journal of Nutrition*, 56(1), 49–58.

Scatliffe, N., Casavant, S., Vittner, D. & Cong, X. (2019) Oxytocin and early parent-infant interactions: a systematic review. *International Journal of Nursing Sciences*, 6(4), 445–53.

Schechtman, V. L., Harper, R. M., Wilson, A. J. & Southall, D. P. (1992) Sleep state organization in normal infants and victims of the sudden infant death syndrome. *Pediatrics*, 89(5 pt 1), 865–70.

Steinman, G. (2001) Mechanisms of twinning. IV. Sex preference and lactation. *Journal of Reproductive Medicine*, 46(11), 1003–7.

Tay, C. C., Glasier, A. F. & McNeilly, A. S. (1996) Twenty-four hour patterns of prolactin secretion during lactation and the relationship to suckling and the resumption of fertility in breast-feeding women. *Human Reproduction*, 11(5), 950–55.

Twins Trust (2020) *BeCOME: Better Care of Multiples – An Exploration.* Aldershot: Twins Trust.

Twins Trust (2021) Neonatal care. Available at http://twinstrust.org/let-us-help/pregnancy-and-birth/in-hospital/neonatal-care.html, accessed 16 September 2022.

Tyson, J. E., Hwang, P., Guyda, H. & Friesen, H. G. (1972) Studies of prolactin secretion in human pregnancy. *American Journal of Obstetrics & Gynecology*, 113(1), 14–20.

UNICEF (2022) How can I tell that breastfeeding is going well? Available at www.unicef.org.uk/babyfriendly/wp-content/uploads/sites/2/2016/10/mothers_breastfeeding_checklist.pdf, accessed 11 May 2022.

Wambach, K. & Spencer, B. (2021) *Breastfeeding and Human Lactation.* 6th ed. Burlington, MA: Jones and Bartlett Learning.

Wiessinger, D., West, D., Smith, L. J. & Pitman, T. (2014) *Sweet Sleep: Nighttime and Naptime Strategies for the Breastfeeding Family.* Raleigh, NC: La Leche League International.

Wilson-Clay, B. (2005) *External Pacing Techniques: Protecting Respiratory Stability during Feeding* [Independent Study Module]. Amarillo, TX: Pharmasoft Publishing.

World Health Organization (2011) Exclusive breastfeeding for six months best for babies everywhere. Available at www.who.int/news/item/15-01-2011-exclusive-breastfeeding-for-six-months-best-for-babies-everywhere, accessed 11 May 2022.

World Health Organization (2021) Complementary feeding. Available at www.who.int/health-topics/complementary-feeding, accessed 11 May 2022.

Yate, Z. M. (2017) A qualitative study on negative emotions triggered by breastfeeding; describing the phenomenon of breastfeeding/nursing aversion and agitation in breastfeeding mothers. *Iranian Journal of Nursing and Midwifery Research*, 22(6), 449–54.

Index